EPILEPSY
Facts about fits

EPILEPSY

Facts about fits

Roy G. Beran

MD, BS, FRACP, FRACGP, FAFPHM, FACLM
BLegS, GradDipTertEd, GradDipFurtherEd

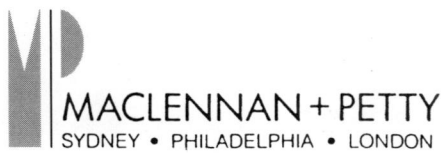

MACLENNAN + PETTY
SYDNEY • PHILADELPHIA • LONDON

First published 1997

MacLennan & Petty Pty Limited
ACN 003 458 973
809 Botany Road, Rosebery, Sydney NSW 2018, Australia

National Library of Australia
Cataloguing-in-Publication data:
Beran, Roy G (Roy Gary).
Epilepsy: Facts about fits
Includes index

ISBN 0 86433 134 7

1. Epilepsy. I. Title
616.853

Printed and bound in Australia

Contents

About the author

Dr Beran is a consultant neurologist who has been in private practice in Sydney, Australia, for more than a decade. His doctoral thesis examined the epidemiology and psycho-social aspects of epilepsy. He has worked as a general practitioner and was formally trained as a teacher and lawyer. He holds appointments, as visiting medical officer in neurology, at Liverpool and Fairfield Hospitals (both teaching hospitals for the University of New South Wales), Royal Rehabilitation Centre (a teaching hospital for Sydney University), Braeside Rehabilitation Hospital, Lachlan Centre (which specialises in caring for those with intellectual challenge) and HMAS Penguin Naval Hospital. He is the consultant in neurology to the Royal Australian Navy and is a visiting fellow to the School of Community Medicine at the University of New South Wales. He has held numerous positions on both the state and federal bodies of the Epilepsy Society of Australia and the National Epilepsy Association of Australia (the national chapters of the International League Against Epilepsy and the International Bureau for Epilepsy). He helped establish the St. Lukes Telemetry Service, the first privately owned video-telemetry service in Australia, at St. Lukes Hospital, and is a foundation member of the neurosciences departments at both St. Lukes and the Mater Hospitals, private hospitals in Sydney. He has trialed new anti-epileptic drugs (in private practice) and has undertaken research in health economics.

Foreword

Few pathological disorders of human function elicit more negative emotional reactions than epilepsy. Throughout history, in almost all cultures, people afflicted with this disorder encountered severe discrimination, perhaps second only to that incurred by leprosy. Epileptic attacks were often viewed as possession by the devil, punishment for sins, evidence of severe psychosis, or a highly contagious disease. Unfortunately, these stigmata have not been completely eradicated by advances of modern biomedical science, and persons with epilepsy and their families still often find it necessary to conceal their affliction out of shame, or the logical desire to avoid the restrictions that society places on individuals who experience sudden losses of control without warning. In most cases, epileptic seizures can now be completely controlled by medication or surgery, but even in the worst conditions the persistent attacks occur relatively infrequently, a few times a week, or perhaps a few times a day, and are usually brief, lasting seconds to but a few minutes. Unless the epilepsy is due to an underlying disorder that also causes neurological or mental disturbances, day-to-day function is likely to be completely normal between seizures. The total time of behavioural epileptic disruption therefore represents an extremely small percentage of the life of a person with epilepsy, but for most the consequent disability is disproportionately great as a result of attitudes of others rather than the disease process itself.

Epilepsy is the most common primary brain disorder, and epileptic seizures are symptoms of a variety of conditions rather than a disease per se. The World Health Organization has recently determined that epilepsy is second only to depression among the central nervous system disorders as a cause of disability worldwide. In recent years, medical science has done much to elucidate the causes of epileptic seizures and to characterise the important features of a variety of epileptic disorders. This has led to safer and more effective modes of treatment, which have resulted in significant reduction or complete elimination of seizures for most patients who suffer from these conditions. Much more needs to be done, however, specifically to alleviate the adverse social consequences of epilepsy. At the present time, the quickest and most cost-effective way to achieve a quantum leap forward in quality of life for patients with epilepsy would more likely come from efforts to eliminate counterproductive societal attitudes than from scientific breakthroughs.

The most important step in addressing stigma and other adverse concepts about epilepsy is education of patients, their family and friends, those with whom they interact on a daily basis (such as employers and teachers), and the public in general. This book is intended for that purpose, and clearly and succinctly translates current scientific concepts of epilepsy into readable lay language. A careful reading of this small volume will do much to dispel myths and misconceptions that plague those who suffer from epileptic seizures, so that the real disabilities can be addressed in a logical and scientific fashion. Dr. Beran is a talented and experienced epileptologist who not only explains this poorly understood and much-maligned illness in easy-to-comprehend terms, but also offers a great deal of wise advice that should be extremely helpful for those who suffer from epilepsy, their families, and everyone who from time-to-time will come into contact with persons with epilepsy and is in a position to influence the impact of this disorder on their lives.

Professor Jerome Engel, Jr., MD, PhD

President, International League Against Epilepsy
Chief, Division of Epilepsy and
Clinical Neurophysiology
Reed Neurological Research Center
University of California, Los Angeles

April, 1997

Preface

This book is intended to help people with epilepsy to understand what epilepsy is and how it may affect them or their family. It is also designed to meet the needs of family physicians, helping to answer the questions that their patients may ask and offering answers in a clear manner to suit both the physicians and their patients.

The text offers many of my personal views. My aim is to create a bond between myself and the reader, whether patient, family member or doctor. I hope readers will be critical and question what is in this book rather than take things at face value. Epilepsy is often referred to as a single 'generic' entity and my earlier research has suggested that its prevalence (the number of cases in the community) may be as high as 1 in 50. The reason my figure was so high was that I looked at something that had not been examined in earlier studies, undertaken in the early 1980s: the number of people who have epilepsy but who refuse to admit to this in scientific research. Up to 1 in 4 people known to have epilepsy (but who did not know that I knew that they had it) denied the diagnosis, thereby suggesting that earlier figures which reported a lower prevalence were probably far too low. For the first time, based on the fact that so many people denied the diagnosis in this research, there was a real indicator of the extent of the perceived stigma felt by those who have epilepsy. The analysis also indicated that epilepsy is more common than had previously been believed and that it is a common condition.

Those who denied the diagnosis of epilepsy made up part of the figure which is called the 'false negative response' rate, representing those not included in the number thought to have the condition, but who should really be counted in. Another cause of false negative response was found by a Polish doctor, Dr Zielinski, who found that 1 in 4 people with epilepsy did not know that they had it because their symptoms of seizures were so mild. This realisation forced me to question what was really meant by the term 'epilepsy' and in reviewing this concept I found new aspects to the broad topic of epilepsy and its management. I was forced to accept that much of what the patient feels and believes about epilepsy is kept totally private from people who research the condition and, at the same time, often things that the expert considers to be part of the picture of epilepsy are considered as quite separate from the diagnosis by the person who has epilepsy.

In a book like this it is only fair to allow you, the reader, to make up your own mind and to help in this process I have made special efforts to highlight those areas within the study of epilepsy (epileptology) where there is room for debate. Prevalence, as described above, is just one of these areas.

In an attempt to give a fair overview of current knowledge I have chosen to emphasise the breadth of present views, but it is impossible to do this without introducing some of my personal bias. Should you find any issues contentious you may wish to drop me a line at my address: **Suite 5, 6th floor, 12 Thomas Street, Chatswood, NSW 2067, Australia.**

After quite some time in private practice as a neurologist I have learnt to listen to alternative views. I realise that such views have often forced me to reconsider many of my own strongly held beliefs. Patients are among my most respected teachers. What they have to say is based on real experiences and it is up to the doctor, in this case me, to explain what my patients tell me, and so learn to understand better what is going on with those patients. I am forced to be critical of what I do and how I do it.

The aim of this book is to help people with epilepsy, their families and friends, cope better with the hassles of day to day living with a condition, that is a source of stigma and negative community attitude. I hope this book will go some of the way to help those affected know what epilepsy is. With more knowledge they may find the commitment to become ambassadors for epileptics. To break down the barriers of ignorance and stigma, people with epilepsy will have to stand up and be counted!

They will have to have the courage to say, 'I'm an epileptic . . . so what! Yes, I'm a person with epilepsy. I have no reason to be ashamed! My epilepsy is not my excuse for what I am. It is my reason for being better, for trying harder and for being proud of overcoming the prejudice that ignorance has generated!'

It is also my aim to help the family doctor better assist patients to deal with their epilepsy and be proud to be ambassadors for epileptics. Family doctors are often expected, unreasonably, to be experts on every condition they encounter. I hope to help them better understand some of the issues involved in epilepsy and its management by sharing the views expressed in this book.

If this simple text achieves only a fraction of my ambitious aims then the effort spent in writing it has been well spent. Please help realise these goals by reading more about epilepsy. Please also take up the offer to write to me and give your views about what this book has to offer and how it can be improved. It is only with feed-back that books such as this can be made more relevant to the needs of their target audience. Thank you for reading on and for being part of my ambitious attempt to improve the material available for people interested in learning about epilepsy.

Chapter 1

What is epilepsy?

Definition

Epilepsy can be defined as a tendency to the recurrence of seizures. Now we need a definition of seizure. Seizures are also called fits, turns, episodes, events, and many people invent 'pet' names for their seizures. In this text the terms 'fits' and 'seizures' will be used interchangeably and the reason for this will be discussed later.

Many texts examine the basis of the word 'seizure', which comes from the Greek word meaning 'to seize'. This adds little to the overall understanding of epilepsy but gives insight to the basis of the stigma attached to it. This stigma relates to the old belief in demonic possession.

A seizure is the body's response to uncontrolled over-activity of part or all of the brain. What happens in a fit is determined by the part of the brain that is affected and how long the seizure lasts. Having stated that epilepsy is a tendency to recurrence of seizures, it follows that, for the definition to apply, a person would need to have had a first fit, then a second fit (to show recurrence) and a third fit (to show a tendency to recurrence). For the condition of epilepsy to be considered, a person must have had at least 3 fits. The next question to be asked is the time frame for the 3 fits. Until recently, if the last fit was more than 5 years ago, then the person has been classed as having inactive epilepsy. Current research has resulted in the shortening of that interval to one year so that if the person has had no fits in the last 12 months then the epilepsy is considered inactive. **If the fits occurred recently (within the last year) then the epilepsy is regarded as active.**

1

Avoid negative concepts in the definition

When giving talks to an audience of people who are not especially well trained in the area of epilepsy, I often start with the
question, 'What is epilepsy?' There will always be someone
who will offer the definition that 'Epilepsy is the result of bad or
altered electricity in the brain'! My response to this suggestion is
to ask, 'How many volts?' This answer is not offered in order to
make a meaningless joke but to emphasise a very important
point that is often overlooked. **When someone is having a major
convulsive seizure they do look like they are being electrocuted.** This can be a very frightening experience for someone
who has never seen a fit. While it is not wrong to say that an
epileptic seizure is the expression of altered brain electricity, it
must be said, and re-said, that the amount of electricity involved
is microvolts (a tiny fraction of a single volt) rather than 240
volts (or the 110 volts of American domestic supply). Hence a fit
poses no immediate risk to anyone who may touch the person
during the seizure.

This can not be stated too forcefully because the idea
of electricity carries with it very negative images and fear.
I am sure that it is these negative images which have contributed
to the stigma that surrounds epilepsy. I do not say this lightly
but ask you to consider the picture, as suggested in the
last paragraph, of someone having a convulsion and I am
confident you will agree that the image you have in your mind's
eye is like that of someone being electrocuted. (Very few people
have actually witnessed anyone being electrocuted, which
of itself adds to the mystique and fear of the unknown.) If you
think back to what you were always taught about electricity I am
sure this recollection will evoke concepts of danger. Children
are taught to stay away from electrical connections because
they are potentially lethal. A combined effect of these fears
and warnings is that if epilepsy is associated with electricity
then the logical consequence is to avoid the person who has
epilepsy. This exaggerated response may have developed on
a totally subconscious level; the outcome is fear, stigma,
avoidance and, for the parent of the child with epilepsy, a great
potential for feelings of guilt. Derived from an unexamined
process, reaction to the person with epilepsy remains
counterproductive.

How the brain works

To help you to understand the idea of tiny electrical currents in the brain, it is worth **explaining how the brain sends its messages from one brain cell to another**. A nerve cell, called a **neurone**, sends its message along its long arm, called the **axon**, to the end of the cell where it then transfers that message to a nearby cell. This sending of the message along the axon is done with a very tiny electrical impulse called an **action potential**, and it is for this reason that the concept of electricity being involved in the fit is actually correct. The electrical impulses generated by nerve cells are not big enough to justify the sort of fear that surrounds the concept of electrocution.

The message is not transferred directly to nearby cells but has to jump a very small gap between the nerve cells. This gap is called the **synapse**, and transfer of the neuronal signal across this gap is made by the release of minute amounts of chemicals called **neurotransmitters**. The effect of neurotransmitters on the nerve is decided by the type of transmitter released. Some transmitters excite the nearby cells. Examples of such excitatory neurotransmitters are glutamate and aspartate. Other transmitters inhibit, or dampen down, the activity of adjoining cells and reduce the activity of these cells. The best known inhibitory neurotransmitter is gamma-amino-butyric-acid (often referred to as GABA).

Some people argue that epilepsy is the brain's expression of imbalance between these excitatory and inhibitory neurotransmitters while others argue that there are faulty connections between the various nerve cells. Another popular theory is that the normal, ordered connections between the neurones have been altered so that one cell sends its message to too many other nerve cells which will then work in harmony with the original messenger cell. This allows these other nerve cells to amplify the activity of this part of the brain, causing the overactivity which is recognised as the seizure.

Fears associated with the definition

The description given above has shown that electrical impulses are involved in the transmission of messages throughout the nervous system but it is important to remember that the amount of electricity is so small as to be of no concern. From the warnings given to children plus the appearance of the person who is having a convulsive seizure, it is easy to understand the development of the wrong idea that epilepsy is both dangerous and contagious. **Epilepsy is not contagious. One cannot catch epilepsy!**

People sometimes use terms like 'brain storms' to describe epilepsy. Some doctors even use pictures of lightening coming out of someone's head to show what happens in a fit. This is a very frightening picture and one that suggests that epilepsy is dangerous to anyone who may be nearby. **It must be stressed that epilepsy is not dangerous to the witness!**

There is a further misconception that because epilepsy comes from the brain it follows that people who have epilepsy must be stupid or cannot think properly. This is not true, but the association of epilepsy and brain damage is real. People who have brain damage, from whatever cause, can also have seizures because the brain damage can alter how the brain works; in such cases it is the brain damage that usually causes the epilepsy rather than the epilepsy causing the brain damage. It must be stated, however, that severe epilepsy can cause damage to the brain if it is allowed to continue for a long time, but this is a rare complication of epilepsy. If fits continue, this state is called **status epilepticus** and will be discussed later.

Emotive terminology

As stated earlier, the terms 'fit' and 'seizure' are being used here to mean the same type of event, which is basically the expression of the epilepsy. This is being done deliberately because often people with epilepsy become upset by the use of words such as 'fit' or 'epileptic' and hold the view that such terms are in some way insulting. It is important that everyone realises that no insult is intended and that attitudes suggesting that insult was intended do very little to ease the situation and just make everyone involved feel uncomfortable.

I have already pointed out that epilepsy, and the thoughts that surround it, can make the person, or their family, feel many negative emotions, of which guilt is perhaps one of the most powerful. People who feel guilt also often feel angry about feeling guilty and want to blame others for making them feel bad. This is particularly so for the parent of the child who has epilepsy. As a parent myself, I can fully empathise with the parents who feel that they have failed a child if that child does not achieve a cherished ambition. How much more easily must this feeling of guilt arise when the child has an illness against which parents can not protect him or her. Added to this is the very real situation in which the parents, family members or acquaintances are subject to the same negative emotions that prevail in the society in which they grew up. This means that people will already hold negative views towards epilepsy. Now the reality of epilepsy in the family forces people into a state of emotional conflict. People cannot always work on the rational plane and emotions such as guilt are not always in their control. In many cases people will not even be aware that the negative feelings are there under the surface and without this understanding will not be able to combat those feelings.

It follows that is very easy to react to terminology such as 'fit' or 'epileptic', shifting anger onto the people who have used these terms. Part of this shift is what doctors call 'projection' because it allows the person to project the blame for these negative emotions onto others and thereby avoid personal feelings of guilt or shame. This reaction only amplifies the anger, creating an impression of being under siege, a feeling of isolation. It is far more constructive to accept that no insult is intended in the use of these terms, to use them as interchangeable with words such as 'seizure', thereby coming to terms with reality. To do this constructively, and willingly, allows people to make that giant step towards acceptance of their own feelings as real and explainable. They can come to terms with their own emotions.

Epilepsy is a very emotive subject and people who have epilepsy, and their families, are caught up in the stigma that surrounds it. They feel that to be called an 'epileptic' is in some way insulting and hence wrong. Again there is the potential for projection of anger or guilt. They fail to see that the person who has low height is short, and the person with a large abdomen is fat, and the person who has diabetes is diabetic and the person with asthma is asthmatic. There is no shame in the person with epilepsy being called an epileptic. 'Epileptic' is a descriptive term and it is only if the person using that term intends insult that offence should be taken. In that situation even a 'politically correct' term would be insulting because that is the intention of the user!

Doctors use the term 'spastic' to mean 'significantly increased muscle tone'; it is a very specific medical term, yet young people in society often use the word as one of insult, meaning that someone is stupid or has mental illness. The answer is not to deride society but rather to educate it. The same educational process needs to be applied to attitudes towards epilepsy. There is nothing to be gained by making others feel guilty about the use of terms such as epileptic but rather we should help them to understand that the epileptic person is just that, a person with epilepsy. This could be forcibly imposed by insisting that terms such as 'fit' and 'epileptic' be no longer used, but that, I would argue, would create resentment amongst those being forced to change their use of language and it would do nothing to change attitudes. It is the attitudes that require revision!

Acceptance of the diagnosis

If the epileptic and family can show that they are above petty grief about a diagnosis, over which there was no control, then others will be prepared to reconsider the position from a positive perspective. The person with epilepsy, their family and friends have the power to change attitudes by standing up and being counted! Because epileptics are upset by the term 'epileptic' they give the message that there is something wrong with being an epileptic. If, on the other hand, they were unconcerned by the label then perhaps the message would be different! It is important to realise that epilepsy is an invisible condition unless a person is having a fit, but the attitude of the person who has epilepsy can be as transparent as the stigma.

Epileptic seizures and epileptic syndromes

The definition of epilepsy is not quite as simple as was suggested in the first paragraph of this chapter. The definition depends upon who is asking the question and the purpose of the question. Experts in the field of epileptology (the study of epilepsy) no longer talk about epilepsy in the singular 'generic' term, but rather they talk about **the epilepsies** or alternatively the **'epileptic syndromes'**. They also talk about **epileptic seizures** which are an important part of epilepsy as they are what people see as the manifestation of the epilepsy and are categorised by a separate classification of their own. The reason for this is that an epileptic syndrome may include more than one epileptic seizure type and, as a result of a consensus between the world experts, through the offices of the International League Against Epilepsy [ILAE] (the international body that represents the professionals — basically the doctors — who specialise in epilepsy), there have emerged internationally accepted classifications so that everyone understands what is meant by the terms used. These classifications, both of the epileptic seizures and of the epilepsies (the epileptic syndromes) will be discussed in Chapter 2.

Epileptology, the study of epilepsy

From the above it can be seen that epilepsy is not a single condition. The study of epilepsy has seen the birth worldwide of a new subspecialty in medicine in general and neurology in particular. In its applications this new subspecialty involves neurologists, general physicians, paediatricians, family doctors, social scientists and people with epilepsy themselves, in the form of self-help groups. The term **epileptology** means the study of epilepsy, and its evolution has seen the coming together of people from around the world combining to undertake research to better understand epilepsy and to improve the well being of epileptics. The aim is one day to conquer this difficult condition that has been around for as long as there has been a documented history of mankind.

To re-emphasise something that was stated earlier, the definition of epilepsy is a tendency to recurrence of seizures and it must be questioned if people who have had only one fit have epilepsy. By definition they do not, because they neither have recurrence nor do they show a tendency to recurrence. On the other hand if the medical history is taken very carefully it will usually be shown that they have had minor episodes of what might be called seizures all their life. In this situation the diagnosis of epilepsy may be totally correct and what was called a single fit is, in reality, just the first recognised fit in a person who has had many unrecognised fits. As stated in the preface, Polish research done in the early 1970s has shown that as many as 1 in 4 people with epilepsy do not know that they have it and have never been to a doctor because of it. This may seem very strange, but all will be explained.

Deja vu (the feeling that the person has done the thing before or has been through the experience before) is the result of a false memory or, alternatively, an uncontrolled overactivity of the memory area of the brain. This is sounding very similar to the description of a seizure, and so it should because a deja vu is a type of fit. This highlights a grey area within the definition because it raises the question, 'If a person has 3 deja vu fits is that person an epileptic?' The definition that has been developed around the significance of recurrence would say, 'Yes'. Obviously this is an impracticable answer because on that basis everyone would be classed as an epileptic. While this is appealing to the person who has epilepsy, and to those who have been angry at being called epileptic, logic dictates that this is not right. Some restrictions need to be placed on the application of the diagnosis or no-one would be allowed to drive a car and everyone would be on anti-epileptic medications.

When to apply the definition

The compromise is to state that the label should only be applied if the seizures are of sufficient severity to significantly interfere with the person's **quality of life**. Even this is not an absolute and there is a need to develop a tool that will allow reproducible measurement of quality of life. Quality of life depends on the culture and expectations of the person involved (not the researcher but the person with epilepsy) because quality of life is a very subjective value judgement and is not something that can be imposed by others. Only the affected person can clearly define the difference between what the person expects from life and what is being realised from life at the time of assessment. The search for an accurate measure of quality of life is becoming one of the most important areas of research in epileptology because it seeks to define one of the basic variables in the measurement of epilepsy, and consequently to assess the value of treatment. In this age of consumerism it is the patient who decides if treatment is adequate.

Again it can be seen that the definition of epilepsy is far from simple. There are different types of fits and different types of epileptic syndromes. In the end the definition of epilepsy is a balance between hard core science and more subjective value judgements. Epileptologists are constantly trying to make a more rigid definition which better allows international comparison of information and from the above it can be seen that they have come a long way in this search, but there is still a long way to go.

Chapter 2

What types of epilepsy are there?

The experts who work in the field of epileptology have developed two different classifications concerning epileptic seizures and syndromes, and at each of the international meetings when these experts come together there is on-going debate to improve and refine the current classifications.

The international classifications were established to set up internationally agreed standards and to make an acceptable tool for both clinical management and research use so that the care provided for patients could be of as high a standard as possible.

The classification of seizures

Epileptic Seizures

Partial Seizures

- Simple Partial Seizures
- Complex Partial Seizures
- Secondarily Generalised Seizures

Generalised Seizures

- Absence Seizures
- Myoclonic Seizures
- Clonic Seizures
- Tonic Seizures
- Tonic/Clonic Seizures
- Atonic Seizures

Unclassifiable Seizures

The classification of seizures, or fits, is based on what happens in the fit and the electroencephalographical features (changes in the brain waves) that accompany the fit. The classification was developed to allow someone who did not actually see the seizure to understand what happened during it and thus be able to compare experiences of people around the world. Unfortunately, an assumption of correct classification is not always justified. A classification is only as good as the classifier.

What happens in a fit is determined by the part of the brain involved in the seizure. A demonstration of this may be found in the type of seizure that results from overactivity of the part of the brain that controls the movement of one of a person's thumbs. As a result of this activity in the brain, the patient will have abnormal uncontrolled movement of the thumb on the side of the body opposite to the side of the brain that is overactive. If this activity spreads on the same side of the brain to involve areas controlling the leg or face, then so will movement in the body spread on the opposite side in what has been called a 'Jacksonian march' (so named to honour Sir Hughlings Jackson, an English neurologist who lived at the turn of the 20th century and described much of what forms the basis for modern epileptology). At this stage within the fit the person may still be alert and conscious as it is only the 'motor' (or movement) part of the brain that is involved in the seizure. If the overactivity in the brain spreads to involve the whole of the brain then the person will lose consciousness and the fit, which started as a simple partial seizure with focal motor expression, will have spread to become a secondarily generalised seizure.

The reason a seizure is called **simple partial** is because it does not cause the person to lose consciousness (that is the meaning of **'simple'** in this classification) and because it started in just one part of the brain. It is important to make the point that when a seizure is called **'partial'** it does not mean that the person has part of a fit but rather that **only part of the brain is involved**. This is also sometimes called **focal**.

As with so many other well meant developments in science, there has emerged a lot of difficulty with some of the terms used in various classifications; people have not understood what was meant. This book aims to remove some of that confusion.

From the patient's point of view, the clinical application of the classification of seizures is by far the most important. As suggested above, epileptic fits are divided into two basic groupings, the partial (focal) seizures and the primarily generalised seizures, which do not show focal onset. There is a third group of seizures which are called unclassifiable seizures because it is impossible to be sure of their basis in type of brain activity and the EEGs are not classic for any of the usual types of seizures.

It is probably unnecessary for the person with epilepsy to learn fully the international classifications and it is probably also true to say that most doctors who treat epileptics do not fully remember the classifications. The original classification of seizures was first published in the late 1960s and, since that time, most doctors have acquired some working knowledge of it and its application, but I am sure that the fine points are not universally understood nor universally applied. The last modification of the classification of seizures was in 1981 and that for syndromes was in 1989, but there is still considerable pressure to revise the classification.

Partial onset seizures

These are focal onset seizures. **The partial seizures are further divided into simple and complex partial seizures plus secondarily generalised seizures.** It is accepted that any of the partial fits can progress from one fit type to another. A person can start with simple partial seizure (in other words, a focal onset fit that is not associated with impairment of consciousness) which then progresses to complex partial seizure (a fit type in which there is impairment of consciousness but the focal nature of the fit is maintained). The fit can progress still further to become a secondarily generalised seizure which is the convulsive conclusion of the spread of brain activity, as was described above. In the secondarily generalised seizure, the focal nature of the fit is replaced by involvement of the whole of the brain at the time of the fit and this causes the person to have a convulsion.

The question of automatism

There is a degree of similarity between the complex partial fit and the type of generalised seizure called absence seizure. In both, the patient is out of contact with the environment, but the complex partial fit is usually followed by a period in which the patient feels strange, confused and tired. In the complex partial seizure there is more likelihood of the patient having what is called an 'automatism'. **An automatism is, as the name implies, characterised by automatic behaviour in which the person has no control over what they are doing.** To the casual observer the person may appear to be in complete control of what he or she is doing but he or she will have no recall of what happened nor remember what he or she did, despite having performed very complex tasks. **Sometimes such automatic behaviour can also occur in generalised absence seizures; these are called complex absence seizures**, and it is most important that the doctor uses the EEG to help decide which type of seizure is being experienced. The importance of deciding which type of fit is being seen is to decide which medicine should be given and this will be discussed later in this book.

People often talk about an '**aura**' preceding the onset of the fit and say that this is the warning that a fit is about to happen. This is not the case! **An aura is a fit**. It is a simple partial seizure in which consciousness is not impaired and there is overactivity in the part of the brain that produces the sensation that is reported as the aura. An example of this is a sensation of the smell of burning rubber in the absence of any rubber being burnt. This represents an overactivity of the part of the brain that is responsible for recording the sensation of smell. Smelling burning rubber prior to the onset of a major convulsive fit is not an aura before a primarily generalised convulsive tonic/clonic fit but rather it is a simple partial fit progressing to a secondarily generalised convulsion.

This subject matter is highly complex, I know. I certainly hope to avoid fuelling confusion, but without acknowledging the complexity of the scope of epileptology there cannot be adequate realisation of the broad range of study that is epileptology and you will not be stimulated to read further. As was stated in the preface, if you have problems with the text, active feed-back is welcome.

Primarily generalised seizures

Primarily generalised fits, fits which are generalised from their onset, are divided into: absence seizures; myoclonic seizures; clonic seizures; tonic seizures; tonic/clonic seizures; and atonic seizures. In each of these fit types there is no definable focal onset to the fit and the EEG, which maps out the brain activity, shows generalised epileptic spike and wave activity from the onset of the fit rather than the focal abnormality which will be found in the partial seizures. Each of these fit types has different features, such as those of the **absence seizure which is the type of epileptic fit that was called 'petit mal' before the use of the new classification** and is described in the section dealing with generalised seizures.

Description of the primarily generalised seizures

As mentioned, the absence seizure was previously referred to as petit mal but this term has been out of vogue for more than 20 years. **The absence seizure** is characterised by the person suddenly stopping what he or she is doing and becoming, as the name implies, mentally absent and out of connection with his or her surroundings. This type of seizure is more common amongst young children. The child may stop, stare, blink the eyes and even nod the head. The fit usually stops as quickly as it starts and the person will be back to normal as soon as the fit stops.

   Myoclonic seizures are fits which are associated with sudden forceful muscle jerks or contractions. The limbs (more commonly the upper limbs) are flung out in a wing-like fashion and the person has no control over this. These fits often occur in the morning, especially if the person has not had enough sleep. A leading Australian epileptologist has called these 'weetie fits' because they are the fits in which the person may have a sudden muscle jerk and as a result fling their weetie (cereal breakfast food) across the room.

Clonic fits cause the person to have repeated muscle spasms but the amount of movement is less dramatic than occurs in myoclonic fits. The repetitive nature of the jerking is more pronounced and of longer duration than in myoclonic seizures.

Tonic fits are associated with sudden spasms of the muscles which may become stiff and project out in front of the person but they lack the violent jerk that is part of the myoclonic episode. People who have tonic fits often fall down as part of the fit and it is sometimes very difficult to tell the difference between tonic and atonic fits. Tonic fits are an important part of the diagnosis of Lennox Gastaut Syndrome (described below).

Tonic/clonic seizures are what most people recognise as epilepsy: they are convulsive episodes and the only question is whether they are primarily or secondarily generalised. It is this type of epileptic fit that was called Grand Mal before the new classifications were accepted.

Atonic seizures occur when the uncontrolled overactivity of the brain causes loss of muscle tone and the person just falls down. In this fit type there is no obvious muscle spasm as was described in tonic fits.

Status epilepticus

If the person has a particularly prolonged seizure or there is little or no time between repeated seizures then these episodes are given another term. This term is **status epilepticus**. The condition of status epilepticus is reason for immediate increased concern and needs professional help. If allowed to continue, status epilepticus can cause death or serious brain damage. **If status epilepticus can be controlled within the first 30 to 60 minutes then the potential damage is usually reversible, but after that time permanent damage and possibly death are quite likely.** Knowing this is to realise the importance of calling for help if a fit lasts any real length of time. The warning bells should be ringing for any fit that lasts for more than 10 minutes because it takes some time to organise things and to stop the fit. Obviously the severity of the potential damage depends upon the fit type. This is of particular relevance to convulsive seizures, rather than non-convulsive seizures, although permanent damage may still result from these minor fit types. The extent of the damage is less clear regarding non-convulsive seizures. Even though brain over-activity complies with the definition of status epilepticus, when this involves non-convulsive seizures the condition may even go unnoticed since the seizure expression can be as trivial as a subtle change in behaviour.

The epileptic syndromes

Epilepsies and Epileptic Syndromes

Localisation-related (focal, local) epilepsies
* *Idiopathic (with age-related onset)*
    Benign childhood epilepsy with centrotemporal spikes
    (benign rolandic epilepsy)
    Childhood epilepsy with occipital paroxysms
    Primary reading epilepsy
* *Symptomatic anatomically and phenomenon defined epilepsies*
    Includes consideration of anatomical onset and seizure type

Generalised epilepsies
* *Idiopathic (with age-related onset)*
    Benign neonatal familial onset
    Benign neonatal convulsions
    Benign myoclonic epilepsy of infancy
    Childhood absence epilepsy (pyknolepsy)
    Juvenile absence epilepsy
    Juvenile myoclonic epilepsy
    Epilepsy with generalised tonic/clonic seizure on awakening

* *Cryptogenic or asymptomatic epilepsies*
    West syndrome
    Lennox Gastaut syndrome
    Epilepsy with myoclonic-astatic seizures*
    Epilepsy with myoclonic absences

* *Symptomatic epilepsies*
    Non-specific aetiology — early myoclonic encephalopathy
    Specific syndromes as accompany other diseases

Epilepsies uncertain if focal or generalised

- *Seizures of illdefined origin*
  Severe myoclonic epilepsy of infancy
  Epilepsy with continuous spike and wave EEG in slow wave sleep
  Acquired epileptic aphasia (Landau-Kleffner syndrome)

Special Syndromes

- *Situation related epilepsies*
  Febrile convulsions
  Isolated seizures or isolated status epilepticus
  Isolated, event provoked, seizures — such as eclampsia, alcohol provoked . . .

[*Astatic seizures are a hangover from an earlier seizure classification and are similar to atonic seizures. Because of the similarity the term does not appear in the current seizure classifications but it remains in the syndrome descriptions.]

The use of the classification of syndromes, rather than that of seizure types, means that the doctor not only knows the type of fit within the type of epilepsy but also understands the natural history of that type of epilepsy. Armed with this knowledge the doctor can give the patient a reliable prognosis and can offer more precise treatment.

Classification of the epilepsies accepts that the first classification, that of the seizures, describes the types of fits but takes this concept one step further and categorises the types of epilepsy or epileptic syndromes in which those fits occur. Some people have found great difficulty in understanding the need for these two different classifications and have felt that the experts are trying to make things so difficult that only an expert can be part of the game.

The above summary of the International Classification of the Epilepsies highlights how complicated the process is. The average reader cannot be expected to become an expert in it, but it is important to recognise that the classification exists and why it exists. As stated earlier, this second classification was needed to try to set out the natural history of the differing types of epilepsies. It is intended to help both doctor and patient understand what to expect from the diagnosis and to help standardise the information used by the specialists who publish scientific papers in the field. The classification has helped doctors around the world compare cases and thus better understand epilepsy in more detail.

It is important to accept and understand the two-tier classification which has now become part of current practice of epileptology. Without this understanding modern literature about epilepsy will be unclear. To study the topic further, as I hope you will, it is important to have a starting point which is clear and concise. The classification of the epilepsies, or the epileptic syndromes, may include more than one type of epileptic seizure in a single type of epilepsy. Thus the second classification depends on the first.

Just as the classification of the seizures was divided into partial and generalised seizures, so too is the classification of the epileptic syndromes divided into localisation-related (and for that read 'focal') and generalised epilepsies. The classification is developed further to try to divide the syndromes on the basis of age of onset, seizure type and causes and structures in the brain that are involved in the seizures. Thus they are divided upon the basis of knowledge of what caused them so that there are 'symptomatic', and 'idiopathic' or 'cryptogenic' subgroupings. 'Symptomatic' epilepsies have a known, identifiable cause while 'cryptogenic' and 'idiopathic' epilepsies do not. The focal epilepsies are also classified according to the part of the brain in which the fit is generated, such as 'Temporal Lobe Epilepsy' or 'Frontal Lobe Epilepsy' in which very specific partial seizures emerge.

Some special subgroups of epilepsies do not really fit into the above groupings and a separate category of epilepsies has been created, called the special or situation related epilepsies. Two appendices have been added to the special category and these appendices include such epilepsies as the reflex epilepsies. Examples are 'reading epilepsy' and 'photo-sensitive' epilepsy.

Detailed knowledge of the classification of epileptic syndromes is really the domain of the doctor, so that the doctor can give the patient advice on what to expect in the future. Once the doctor has defined the seizure type, the duration of the fit, the predominant time of occurrence, the frequency and the activation pattern, then the next step is to define the part of the brain that is involved. If the doctor can add to this an understanding of the cause of the fits and possibly even the genetic predisposition, based on the family history, then there should be enough information to give the patient a recognised syndromic name to identify the type of epilepsy that the person has.

The experts recognise that one syndrome type can progress to another in much the same way that there can be progression through the partial seizures (with simple partial seizures becoming secondarily generalised). This recognition has developed with the use of increasingly sophisticated technology. One subgroup affected by this development is idiopathic or cryptogenic localisation-related epilepsy. This term can be simplified to read 'epilepsy with a focal seizure pattern for which no cause has been determined'. This classification of a particular type of syndrome may have been correct for a particular patient before the doctor had access to more sophisticated scanning techniques which are discussed in later chapters. Once better scanning was available then a cause for the epilepsy may have been found and the old classification therefore no longer considered correct. Our understanding of the causes of epilepsy has improved greatly, especially with better imaging, and it should not be seen as a criticism of the doctor to recognise that this has resulted in altered classification.

Much of what has been set out in this chapter will become clearer as you move further into this book, but for now the following will offer a simple stepwise method of classifying a particular patient according to the international guidelines.

Logical progression and application of the classifications

LEVEL 1: Seizure classification based on history and description of the fit, physical examination, investigation (especially EEG) and review

LEVEL 2: Lateralisation or localisation of the fit onset using the latest technology (a situation that is constantly changing and improving)

LEVEL 3: Definition of cause of the epilepsy (e.g. special type of inherited illness or brain condition)

LEVEL 4: Syndromal classification according to the knowledge and understanding that is available at the time of classification

Examples of a syndrome

To help solidify the complex concept of the classification of the epilepsies, what will follow is a number of examples of different types of epilepsy so that you will appreciate the need to have two different classifications. I hope that the combination of these examples, plus the above stepwise progression, will bring an end to the confusion, but if there remain questions to be answered please refer to the Preface and contact me directly.

Description of one of the epilepsies may help in the understanding of the syndromes. The **Lennox Gastaut Syndrome** occurs more commonly in children but does also occur in adults. It includes generalised tonic seizures, myoclonic seizures, tonic/clonic seizures and may also include atonic seizures plus both simple absence and atypical absence seizures. It is associated with a special electroencephalographic (EEG) pattern of slow spike and wave brain discharges. The person who has it is usually very difficult to treat, is intellectually impaired with developmental delay, and has a poor prognosis. It can be seen that the use of this term is specific and the reader who understands the term knows exactly what is meant (assuming that the person who uses the term is using it correctly).

Another type of epileptic syndrome is **Juvenile Myoclonic Epilepsy**, a type of generalised epilepsy characterised by myoclonic fits which are particularly prone to occur if the person has had late nights, has drunk too much alcohol or has failed to be compliant with medication. These patients often only present after they have had their first major convulsive seizure and it is only then, after the doctor takes a detailed history, that it emerges that they have had myoclonic fits for years. Interestingly enough, the patients often have dismissed these early morning myoclonic fits as early waking clumsiness, further testimony to the report set out in the preface in which it was stated that many people with epilepsy are unaware that they have it.

To conclude this chapter I will describe just one more type of epilepsy, **Frontal Lobe Epilepsy**. This is a particular type of focal, anatomically defined epilepsy in which the patient may show the very bizarre behaviour to be expected from someone with damage to the frontal lobe. The frontal lobe is the part of the brain which provides us with inhibitions that modify our behaviour in daily life. These patients often display provocative sensual, sexual activity during their fits and may be accused of having pseudoseizures (which are not real fits but are discussed in Chapter 7 in the section dealing with seizure look-alikes). It is important to be aware of this type of epilepsy because the possibility of dismissing it as something other than epilepsy is very high.

Chapter 3

How is epilepsy diagnosed?

The diagnosis of epilepsy is not always as easy as one might think. It has already been shown that the definition of epilepsy can be quite difficult and what seemed easy at the introduction to Chapter 1 became far less clear by the end of that chapter.

History is most important

Some types of epilepsy are very easy to diagnose. It is very easy to diagnose epilepsy in a person in whom one has seen a major convulsive fit and of whom there is a clear eye witness report of at least 2 other such convulsive seizures. This is not where the problem arises. The problem occurs when the history is more subtle. In some cases the diagnosis will be more speculative. In some cases the doctor will say, '. . . I think this person has epilepsy, but I'm not sure . . .' There may be need for a subspecialist or expert to be involved in making the diagnosis and even then the diagnosis will not always be one hundred per cent certain.

If the history is absolutely convincing then the diagnosis is confirmed even if every test is negative. **No test can undo what an absolute history of definite seizures puts in place.** There are a number of things that can be mistaken for epilepsy. Just some of them will be discussed now to show what is meant.

Some of the things that can be confused with epilepsy include: a faint (also called syncope); breath-holding attacks in children; or even daydreaming (which may be confused with absence seizures).

The doctor should take as crisp and exact a history as is possible. Often patients will say that they do not know what happened to them. While this may be true to some degree it is never completely true. A person will know how he or she felt before the episode, if the tongue was bitten or if urine or faeces were passed during the particular episode under review. Patients will be able to tell if they were confused, had a headache or were sleepy after the event.

You will, hopefully, have noted that the term seizure, or fit, has been carefully avoided in the preceding paragraph. This has been done deliberately because it is vital that the doctor does not jump to conclusions. **It is far easier to give a person the diagnosis or label of epilepsy than it is to remove it!** It is therefore most important that the doctor only labels reported episodes as epileptic, or as fits, when the diagnostic process has been exhausted and diagnosis is in no doubt.

In some cases, even the most detailed history will not give an absolute diagnosis and there will be a need to get extra information. Eye witness accounts often help in the diagnosis of epilepsy but they do not always give the final answer and at times can be quite confusing. To witness a loved one having a convulsion, or even something that is wrongly thought to be a convulsion, can be very frightening. In such a situation the description may be vague or even, at times, completely wrong and misleading. The doctor always has to question what is being said and if in doubt must take the matter further. One way of doing this is to admit the person to a hospital or centre where prolonged video-telemetry is available. This will be discussed in more detail later but for now it is enough to say that this procedure allows the doctor to video record both what the person does in a fit, assuming that a fit happens, and the brain activity at the time of the video recording.

The role of the electroencephalograph (EEG)

If the history is totally convincing one could argue that there is no need to go further, though very few doctors would not do an electroencephalograph (EEG) even in such a case. An EEG records the small discharges which represent the activity of the brain. Just as a cardiograph (ECG) records the activity of the heart and gives an idea of what is happening in the heart, so the EEG gives an idea of what and where things are happening in the brain. If the doctor and patient are lucky, the EEG will record a fit but this is rarely the case. If a fit is recorded then this will give absolute confirmation of the diagnosis and make the doctor's job so much easier, especially if the history is only suggestive rather than diagnostic of epilepsy. It must be accepted that a normal EEG does not exclude the diagnosis of epilepsy and so the doctor does everything possible to help the patient have a fit at the time of recording.

Those things known to provoke a fit are the things that the doctor will ask the patient to do to increase the likelihood of obtaining a positive EEG. Such things include sleep deprivation and the doctor may ask the patient to stay awake for anything up to three days. Usually, if three days without sleep is required, the patient will be admitted into hospital. A one to two day sleep deprivation EEG will often be done with the patient at home and the family helping to keep the patient awake. Sleep deprivation causes people to be fatigued, cranky and upset and will allow a patient to fall into natural sleep during the recording. Unfortunately most of the drugs which help people sleep have a direct effect on the EEG and thus are of little help in getting more information from the EEG study. The person needs to be naturally tired and to have natural sleep; hence the need for sleep deprivation.

Other things known to increase the yield of the EEG include heavy breathing (also called hyperventilation or overbreathing) and the EEG technician will ask the patient to do this for approximately three minutes during the recording of the EEG. Opening and closing the eyes can also increase the yield as can the use of flashing strobe lighting and most studies will include these two things.

Sometimes none of these will be enough to get a positive study and then the doctor may use video-EEG (referred to earlier). The patient is connected to EEG equipment at the same time as being kept under observation with video recording, so that the doctor can see the brain activity as well as what the patient is doing at the time of any recorded fit. This is also called video-telemetry because it sends the signals to a recording station which may be in a room apart from the patient. The technician or nurse can observe the patient from a remote location by transmitted signals sent by either 'hard wire' recording (where the signal is transmitted along 'wire' cables) or by radio waves. This allows the person to be in as natural an environment as the particular setting which houses the telemetry unit will allow. This is not always as 'user friendly' as one might wish it to be and is subject to the costs which always limit the availability of optimal health care. Some centres only perform daytime, 8-hour, video-telemetry. Other centres allow the patient to be admitted to hospital for as long as it takes to record sufficient fits for the doctor to be confident that the patient either has, or has not, got epilepsy. Video-telemetry is also used if the patient is being considered for epilepsy surgery as it helps to find the site from which the epilepsy is being generated, but this is another story and will be discussed later.

Sometimes the video-telemetry will also have a therapeutic benefit as the doctor can show the recording to the patient and the patient's family. This will allow eye witnesses to confirm that what the doctor recorded is in fact what the eye witness was reporting as a fit. By this use of video, the diagnosis can be either confirmed or excluded. It can also be used to show patients what they do in a fit. This might help them to come to terms with the diagnosis and possibly to realise that it is not as bad as they thought. Ignorance leads to fear of the unknown and use of video-telemetry carries with it extra benefit from showing this unknown.

Discussion of epilepsy and EEG would not be complete without touching on the role of depth electrodes and other sophisticated EEG investigations. These techniques are used when the doctor is trying to decide exactly where within the brain the epilepsy starts. This is vital information when epilepsy surgery is contemplated. The doctor may use electrodes, placed inside the substance of the brain, in the area where the epilepsy is thought to start and video-telemetry is used to record both the epileptic activity inside the brain and what the person does in the fit. Other types of EEG are also sometimes used, such as those obtained when strip electrodes are placed outside the substance of the brain but inside the calvarium (the box that is the brain box — the head). This is just another technique used to determine the site in the brain of the origin of the epileptic activity.

Magnetic encephalograph (MEG)

Tools to measure brain activity are improving and there is a new form of encephalograph called magnetic encephalograph (MEG). This does not measure the tiny electrical impulses as measured by the EEG, but measures the tiny magnetic fields that go with the brain's activity. The MEG is still a research tool but the aim of this book is to introduce new ideas and tools to encourage further reading. MEG is basically only used in the area of epilepsy surgery and is only available in very few centres.

The need for further investigations

By now the doctor should have enough information to either make or break the diagnosis of epilepsy and/or at least give the patient a high degree of reliability regarding the diagnosis. In some people even all the investigations mentioned may not give an absolute diagnosis but in such cases nothing else will and both patient and doctor will just have wait till the illness declares itself in more detail.

The analysis of the patient's condition does not stop here. **The diagnosis of epilepsy is not enough — the doctor must also try to find out why the person has epilepsy!**

Chapter 4

How is epilepsy investigated?

The doctor needs to try to go further than just diagnosing epilepsy as a broad category. The seizure type needs to be defined, and even then there is still a need to establish the syndrome involved. To diagnose just as epilepsy is like saying that an infection is present — such a diagnosis only goes part of the way in helping to treat what is wrong. With an infection the doctor needs to find out what type of infection the patient has so that the best treatment can be given. Similarly the doctor needs to find out what type of epilepsy the patient has, and even more importantly the doctor needs to work out, if possible, why the person has epilepsy. If this is known the doctor can decide how best to treat not only the fits but also the cause of the seizures. Only with all this information can the doctor offer the patient optimal care and give some idea of what to expect for the future (the prognosis).

The need for correct classification

With greater availability of a wider range of newly developed anti-epileptic medications it has become even more important to categorise the patient into the ILAE classifications so that appropriate decisions can be made. **Doctors try to match the fit type with the medication which is thought to best treat it.** Examples of this matching are the use of sodium valproate for myoclonic seizures or the use of carbamazepine for complex partial seizures. Medications and their role in the treatment of epilepsy will be discussed later in this book but for now the point has been made that it is important to know what type of fit is experienced so as to give optimal treatment.

Just as the person who has an infection wants to know what to expect for the future, so the epileptic, or his or her family, wants to know what the future holds. Part of the answer to this question is found in clear definition of the epileptic syndromes. For example, Lennox Gastaut Syndrome, as described in Chapter 2, is known to have a poor prognosis. On the other hand, Juvenile Myoclonic Epilepsy, also described in Chapter 2, responds very well to the use of sodium valproate, plus a change in lifestyle which ensures that the person gets sufficient sleep and does not drink too much alcohol. Juvenile Myoclonic Epilepsy has a good prognosis.

The role of cerebral imaging

The answer to why a person has seizures requires further investigation. This is particularly so if the person had a focal abnormality on the EEG. The doctor needs to find out what has caused this focal change and if there is a lesion (structural abnormality) in the brain which can be treated. To do this the doctor will want to know what the brain looks like. The next step will depend on the level of sophistication available to the doctor and the type of imaging tool at the doctor's disposal.

Skull X-rays are no longer of great benefit in looking at what is going on inside the head and are no longer used in epilepsy assessment except in fairly primitive environments in which this is the only tool available. In these settings it is still of some value to know if there is calcification within the brain but, with better imaging available, new techniques help to go further and give some idea what the nature of the abnormality is and how to treat it.

Computerised tomography (CT)

Most centres now have access to a computerised tomographic scan (CT). This uses X-rays plus sophisticated computer technology to produce much more detailed images of what the organs look like and it gives an idea of the anatomy of the structures in the head. Modern CT uses special equipment and rapid data acquisition to give very detailed pictures that can even do CT scanning on moving patients and hence have a role in the assessment of intellectually handicapped patients. For these patients there has developed 'politically correct' terminology. One of the terms used is 'developmentally delayed', also referred to as 'DD', and more recently the term 'intellectually challenged' seems to be gaining favour. Just as the debate regarding 'epileptic' as compared with 'person with epilepsy' is counter productive for the purposes of this book, so I will dwell no longer on the debate concerning the latest terminology for DD. These patients form a large part of any specialist epilepsy practice and anything that can help in the assessment of them is a boon. No offence is intended by the terminology used.

The latest technology, using special Spiral CT with new software programming, allows the radiologist (X-ray specialist) to perform angiography, mapping out the blood vessels inside the head. This can now be done without the need for passing tubes (catheters) through the blood vessels, a procedure which has the risk of causing a stroke. Angiography has value if the doctor wants to know if there is an aneurysm, a ballooning of the weakened walls of a blood vessel. An aneurysm may cause a bleed inside the patient's head which in turn can cause a fit. This type of CT and its blood vessel imaging is called CTA. The procedure is not available everywhere although there are enough done to merit a mention in this book.

Even CT is losing favour amongst epileptologists because CT misses many of the more subtle abnormalities such as damage to the hippocampus (a part of the brain that is often found to be damaged in patients with temporal lobe epilepsy). CT may also miss 'migration abnormalities', which are special problems with the development of the brain such that the wrong, or abnormal, tissue appears in the wrong places in the brain.

Magnetic resonance imaging (MRI)

Some tumours are also missed on CT and thus **doctors now favour the use of magnetic resonance imaging** (a technique that uses large powered magnetic fields to produce photographic images of the brain by means of special computer technology and recording procedures) [MRI]. It is very similar to CT as far as the patient is concerned. The person lies on a 'table' with a moving top and moves into a tube where the MRI machine records the information to make the pictures. It is not a painful investigation but the tube is quite tight and the MRI is quite noisy. This means that it can be a frightening investigation for people who suffer with fear of confined places (claustrophobia).

The images produced by MRI are far more detailed than those produced by CT and so where doctors have access to MRI they prefer this to CT. MRI is also being constantly improved so that it is now possible to perform what is called **MRI spectroscopy**, a technique available in only very few centres. This tool gives some insight into the brain's functional activity. Previous MRI only gave anatomical pictures but this new use shows how the brain works. It is still very much a research tool but may have wide application in the future.

Just as with CTA, there is also the capacity for MR Angiography [MRA] in which the MRI can be used to image the blood vessels in the head without the need for catheterisation and the increased risk of stroke. This technique is less widely available than is CTA, because MRI is less available than CT, but, depending on which blood vessels are to be imaged, the pictures of the vessels will be better using one of these techniques and cause far fewer risks for the patient. It is worthwhile discussing the choice of imaging with the radiologist before ordering a test as the field of imaging is becoming so sophisticated that it takes an expert's opinion to choose the right test in the right situation.

Unfortunately MRI is not universally available and is quite costly. Not every doctor who works in epileptology has the luxury of MRI and there are two levels of patient care emerging. This is even further emphasised with the addition of some of the new nuclear medicine imaging techniques. These include single photon emission computer tomographic (SPECT) scanning and positron emission tomographic (PET) scanning which are only available in specialised centres. In a country the size of Australia there are only two PET scanners and even these are of differing levels of sophistication.

Positron emission tomography (PET)

PET uses a medical cyclotron (a machine which makes radioactive compounds) to make short half-life isotopes (radioactive compounds) that are too unstable to be taken to centres away from the immediate place housing the cyclotron; they break down too quickly. The isotope chemically binds to everyday compounds that the body (or in the case of epilepsy research — the brain) metabolises and allows the researcher to measure how the person metabolises these everyday substances. **It must be understood that the amount of nuclear irradiation involved is minute and should not cause unnecessary fear for the patient.** The imaging equipment must be next to the cyclotron so that the radioactive substances can be injected into the patient as soon as possible, because, as said above, these substances have such a short half-life. The term **'half-life' refers to the time taken for a compound to be reduced to half the original amount and is used in both nuclear medicine and pharmacology where doctors talk about the half-life of drugs in the body (namely, the time the body takes to reduce the amount of drug to half what was given).** This technique allows the doctor to get pictures of how the brain metabolises such compounds and thus gives pictures of the way the brain works rather than just the anatomy of the brain. It can be seen that PET and functional MRI perform similar tasks and the final role of each of these tools has not yet been defined.

PET can also map out the places in the brain to which certain compounds and drugs may attach. (These are called receptor sites because they have areas in their structure which recognise and link to the compounds to which they bind.) The costs and lack of availability of PET make it only a research tool but it has greatly helped in our understanding of epilepsy and has been used to better locate the origin of the epilepsy in patients being considered for epilepsy surgery, something that will be discussed later.

Single photon emission computerised tomography (SPECT)

SPECT is more freely available than PET but it is still not universally available to all doctors and is still considered by many to be only a research tool. SPECT also uses nuclear technology but uses chemicals that are more stable than those used in PET and thus does not need a medical cyclotron at the same place as the camera which images the patient. It still requires a sophisticated nuclear medicine department or private practice, equipped with the special cameras needed to record the pictures of the brain that are produced by this technique. SPECT is usually used to map the way the brain uses blood. It is thought that, if parts of the brain are using more blood to meet their needs, it can be assumed that these parts of the brain are more active at the time of scanning. It can be seen that both SPECT and PET examine brain function and this changes at the time of the fit. The part of the brain that is the focus of the epilepsy is usually less active at times between fits and becomes more active at the time when fits occur. SPECT is also being used to record receptor sites. Its application to the understanding of epileptology is constantly expanding but still remains within the area of research.

The choice of imaging

The doctor will use whatever imaging tools are available and with which he or she is comfortable. Use of these tools may show what damage (if any) there is in the brain and the nature of that damage will determine the next step in the management of the patient. Many of the abnormalities that have come to light since the advent of MRI are of academic interest only and cannot be treated. Examples are the definition of brain damage that has been present since birth, or developmental abnormalities such as abnormal brain cell migration patterns that cannot be changed. Just because these findings cannot be treated does not mean that the doctor should stop looking for them. Only with our increased knowledge of what is present can we better understand the nature of the epilepsy and what causes it. It only seems like yesterday when doctors said that most forms of epilepsy were idiopathic (conditions for which the cause is unknown) and now it seems that most epilepsy can be traced to a cause of sorts.

The purpose of brain imaging is to look for causes of the epilepsy that can be treated and it is the duty of the doctor to define these and to treat them accordingly. Relevant abnormalities include brain abscesses, tumours and abnormal collections of blood vessels known as arteriovenous malformations. It is most important to diagnose these so that they can be treated surgically if this is possible. Where there is evidence of brain damage without another abnormality such as those listed above, it is still important to identify the damaged area in the brain because, in some cases of difficult-to-manage epilepsy, it may be possible to remove the damaged part of the brain and in so doing stop the fits happening. This is epilepsy surgery and will be discussed in Chapter 8.

Physical examination is mandatory

Investigation of the patient does not stop with EEG and brain imaging. The need for a detailed medical examination of the patient at the time of initial presentation has not been fully emphasised. This is basically because, in the bulk of patients presenting with epilepsy, usually no abnormality will be found. This does not mean that the doctor can bypass the need to examine patients. Sometimes abnormalities will be found that clearly change the approach to managing the case. It should not be ignored that in some cases alternative diagnosis may be found as a result of physical examination or even from the EEG recording [which should include in its detail an ECG (cardiograph) rhythm strip]. Maybe a cardiac cause of loss of consciousness may be detected from heart examination as a result of the initial assessment.

One should never lose sight of the fact that not everyone who presents with suspected seizures has epilepsy and other diagnoses need to be considered. Hence **physical examination is most important** to ensure that the correct diagnosis is made as well as ensuring that concomitant epilepsy diagnoses are also investigated correctly.

Physical examination is also important in a variety of illnesses that have epilepsy as part of their picture. Such conditions include neurofibromatosis which may show 'café au lait' spots. These are, as the name implies, skin areas that are the colour of milk coffee and if the person has six of these, or even just one really large one, then the diagnosis of this condition is made. Sometimes the doctor may have overlooked the presence of such skin lesions and it may help everyone if the patient who knows they are there brings them to the attention of the doctor. Neurofibromatosis is dominantly inherited; with its diagnosis comes the advantage of knowing that 50% of the patient's offspring can be expected to have the condition. Other skin lesions may also have significance, such as blood coloured skin lesions that may alert the doctor to the possible presence of similar lesions in the brain. This condition is known as Sturge Weber Syndrome and includes facial and cerebral angiomata (abnormal collections of blood vessels). **The need for a good medical examination cannot be over-stressed.**

The need for other investigations

The doctor will also want to do blood tests to look for other conditions, such as diabetes or electrolyte disturbances, which can cause seizures. Infections can cause fits, especially in children and blood cultures may therefore sometimes be required. **The doctor may wish to look for infective agents, in the cerebrospinal fluid (often just called the CSF), the fluid that bathes the brain. For this investigation the doctor will need to do a lumbar puncture (also called a spinal tap or abbreviated to LP).** Specimens from the lumbar puncture will be sent to a laboratory to be looked at under a microscope and also sent for culture to try to grow the organism causing any infection. Often, even when there is an infection, the doctor is not able to grow the agent causing it but the tests still need to be done, especially for children.

In some cases other drugs or alcohol may have caused the fits and the doctor may want to look for these. These investigations may need either blood or urine tests. Sometimes the doctor may think that the epilepsy is related to infections in the urinary tract, especially in females. This possibility is of particular significance in those with intellectual problems for whom a history is impossible to obtain. Thus there are a number of reasons why **the doctor may wish to do urine tests** in the epileptic patient.

The above list is not considered to be exhaustive but it does show that the **doctor needs to do quite a number of tests to look for the cause of the epilepsy even after the diagnosis of epilepsy**

has been established and confirmed. Yet again it can be seen that investigation for epilepsy is not as straightforward as was originally thought. The need for expert involvement is re-emphasised as a way of ensuring that uncommon problems are identified and difficulties avoided.

Chapter 5

What should you do when someone has a fit?

The right thing to do during a seizure is determined by the type of fit that the person is having and whether the person having the fit is known to have epilepsy. This may sound somewhat obtuse but it is important. The approach is different in the case of a seizure in a known epileptic to a case where the person is not known to be epileptic. Obviously if the person is known to have epilepsy then it follows that he or she will have been assessed and should already be on treatment. Much of the preliminary ground work will have been completed and need not be repeated. It is necessary to check that this is the case and to review the results of the earlier investigations. You should never lose sight of the first and unchanging rule of good medical practice: trust no one.

Usually the question 'What should you do when someone has a fit?' assumes that the situation is one of major tonic/clonic convulsive seizure. Obviously the question derives from the usual error of assuming that epilepsy is a single 'generic' sickness. You already know that this is not the case and what follows will examine what to do in a variety of seizure types.

What should you do if witnessing a convulsion?

This question has been carefully worded. It makes no value judgement as to the nature of the convulsion, nor does it try to diagnose the illness that has led to the convulsion.

The most important thing to remember is to **protect the person from harm**. If the person having the convulsion is in

36

danger of harm from broken glass or other objects such as sharp-edged furniture, or if he or she is close to stairs or in traffic on the road, then the first rule should be to remove what danger can be removed and warn other people to keep back. Once protective action has been taken then attention should be focused on the person who is convulsing.

Above all else it is important to **remain calm and don't panic**. It may help to know that the person having the convulsion does not know what is happening and that it is only the witness who is frightened. **At the time of the convulsion the person having it is not aware of anything and is in no pain.**

Witnessing a seizure makes the witness feel impotent and useless because as a rule, short of administering medications, there is nothing that can be done to stop a fit. **However, if a fit lasts more than 10 minutes it should be treated as a medical emergency because there is then the worry of status epilepticus.** Unless you know that the person always has 10-minute fits it is worthwhile calling an ambulance when witness to a prolonged fit because status epilepticus is potentially a life threatening illness, especially if the fit lasts more than half an hour. After about half an hour of fitting there is a real risk of permanent brain damage. Usually a fit only lasts one or two minutes and in this case there is no need to call an ambulance unless there is some other form of complication.

The person in the convulsion should be placed in the coma position, lying on their side with their head turned to the side. This will protect him or her from aspirating (breathing in) any vomit if vomiting has occurred during the fit. The coma position protects the lungs. Other than placing the person in this position you should not try to restrain the person. Unless the situation places a person at risk, and that has already been discussed, then he or she will not suffer harm during the clonic, or shaking, part of the seizure. There is nothing to be gained by stopping the person moving about during the clonic period. There is a type of epilepsy known as frontal lobe epilepsy, described in Chapter 2, where the person may thrash about, and in this type of epilepsy you should only consider restraint if the person is at risk of harm because of the situation surrounding the fit. **Common sense must dictate what needs to be done.**

If you are present at the time of a fit you should **loosen tight**

clothing, such as a neck tie, and if possible, without causing harm, **remove foreign objects such as false teeth or food from the person's mouth.** It is most important not to force anything into the person's mouth. **A person having a convulsion cannot swallow his or her tongue and the helper will only risk doing harm by forcing something between the teeth if the person is still in the spasm or tonic phase of the fit.**

In most situations the fit will only last one or two minutes and there will be no need to call for immediate help. Nor is there usually a need to do any more than provide commonsense first aid. Once the person has regained consciousness it is helpful to tell them what has happened and to offer reassurance that he or she is safe and that all is well. At this time it is important to **find out if he or she is known to have epilepsy and if so what type of epilepsy.** It is important to know if the fit just experienced was the same as other usual fits because **if it was not then there is a need to encourage medical review** to investigate the change. It is also important to **find out if the person is on medications and if so what medications**, because the commonest cause for fitting in a person known to have epilepsy is forgetting to take medications. It may be helpful to make sure that if medication has been forgotten a dose is taken as soon as possible.

In the introduction to this section, the point was made that **it is wrong to automatically assume that what seemed to be an epileptic seizure was indeed an epileptic seizure. It may have been a heart attack or the person may be a diabetic** and the episode, while appearing to be epileptic, may have represented a diabetic hypoglycaemic (low blood sugar) event. Hence it is important to ask about past medical history once the person has come out of the convulsion. Often the person will be confused and disorientated after the fit and may be in need of comforting and reassurance.

If the person is slow to come out of the fit, it may be necessary to have a look at their personal belongings. He or she may carry some form of identifying information, such as an identifying bracelet or a card in their wallet. For self-protection, it may be advisable to have someone as a witness while you go through the person's belongings, especially purse or wallet, so that you are not accused of stealing after he or she comes back to normal. **If the person is not known to have epilepsy and this**

is a first convulsion then it is wise to insist on medical attention even in the face of resistance. In this situation it is wise to call an ambulance because, if still in the post-ictal (after the fit) confusional state, a person may be unable to judge what is the correct thing to do and therefore resist good advice.

If the person is known to have epilepsy then there may be no need for anyone to do any more than make sure that he or she knows what happened and is now back under self-control. Again commonsense must dictate what needs to be done at this time.

What should you do if witnessing a non-convulsive seizure?

Often you will not realise that a person is having a seizure if there is no associated convulsion. The person may just seem to be vague or to be behaving in a strange manner. In most such situations the witness is not welcome and others may even assume that the person having the fit is mad or under the influence of alcohol or other drugs. It is only with a high index of suspicion or prior knowledge that the witness will recognise what is happening as a fit.

If the person is known to have this type of epilepsy then all that is required is to **make sure that the person is safe.** This is particularly important with people who are prone to automatisms (automatic behaviour over which they have no control) because they may place themselves in dangerous situations such as walking out in front of cars on a busy road or moving out in front of an oncoming train. It is worth keeping an eye on someone who is acting in a strange fashion because he or she may suddenly change behaviour and for no reason come back to a normal behaviour. If this happens then epilepsy should always be considered as a possible cause for what was thought to be the abnormal behaviour. In this situation all you can do is voice this concern to the person involved and hope that he or she will seek medical attention.

Often it is the teacher at school who first notices that a child is prone to day dreaming or other abnormal behaviour in the class and brings this to the attention of parents who may or may not be prepared to listen and take the child to the doctor. It is consoling to think that even if the person seems to ignore timely advice it may be repeated later by others and it may be just because the advice is repeated that the person ultimately goes to the doctor. Hence you should not be too despondent if a person, or the family, ignore the initial suggestion, even though it is given for good reason and with high probability of being sound. You can never be responsible for the actions of others, but you need to know that you have acted in good faith, in the correct fashion and more cannot be done. **You cannot force someone to seek medical attention unless he or she is a danger to self or others and that is sometimes hard to prove.**

Is there anything else you should do?

There are two other things that are advisable for the witness to a seizure to do. The first relates to the last paragraph, which addresses the question of what to do if the person refuses help and the witness is convinced that help is required. You can always call for an ambulance if you see a person behaving in an exceptionally strange fashion. **It is not only epilepsy that can cause a person to behave in a strange manner!** Other causes of strange behaviour include frank psychiatric illness, diabetic hypoglycaemia (too little sugar in the blood) or even hyperglycaemia (too much sugar in the blood), or various drugs (such as LSD or hallucinogens), or even some food stuffs (like mushrooms). In these situations, a person may need medical attention as a matter of urgency and **not to call an ambulance could be a very wrong decision.**

If you cannot call an ambulance but feel that the person is in need of help, then **you can always turn to the police**, who are trained in first aid and may have the power to insist on medical attention being provided. In any case it is wrong to ignore a situation if you feel that something needs to be done as a matter of urgency and the above approach allows you to leave the scene knowing that you have done all that can be expected from an 'innocent by stander'.

The other important and necessary thing is to document what happened in the fit! Once all required first aid measures have been taken, then it is extremely helpful for the witness to **write**

down exactly what was seen during the fit. In the section dealing with diagnosis, the point was made that there is no more valuable tool with which to make a diagnosis than a clear and explicit history. **There is nothing more important in that history than an eye-witness account** of what happened during a fit. This may be the first time that a reliable eye-witness can actually describe the fit and it would be irresponsible for such a witness not to make notes of what happened. Copies of these notes should be given to the person to show to the doctor. **Such notes could make or break the diagnosis of epilepsy.**

Chapter 6

What causes epilepsy?

Much of what was said in Chapter 4 about necessary tests also gave an idea of what causes epilepsy. As said earlier, the doctor does tests to find treatable causes of the epilepsy but it must be remembered that not all causes of epilepsy are treatable!

The inheritance of epilepsy made simple?

One of the first questions that people ask about epilepsy is if it is inherited. The simple answer is 'Yes!', but, like many viewpoints described in this book, this is not the full answer and it is not as simple a question as it first may have seemed.

Some forms of epilepsy are quite definitely inherited. Most of the primarily generalised forms of seizures have a very obvious familial pattern and are inherited with a dominant type of inheritance. It almost seems as though every day there is reported the discovery, based on well documented family trees and the application of fairly standard genetic laws, of yet another type of dominantly inherited epilepsy. This means that in such cases 50% of the children of an epileptic parent can be expected to have the condition. (Dominant inheritance is discussed below.)

Epilepsy is associated with a number of medical conditions which of themselves are subject to defined patterns of inheritance. An example is the condition called tuberous sclerosis (a condition that will not be further discussed here other than to say that amongst other manifestations of this illness are lesions, inside the brain, which are calcified and hence can act as focal points for fits). Tuberous sclerosis is dominantly inherited and is associated with fits and so it follows that the epilepsy associated with this condition is also inherited as a dominant form of epilepsy. Neurofibromatosis, discussed in Chapter 4, is another condition which is dominantly inherited and also has epilepsy as part of its picture.

In the circumstance of dominant inheritance, the affected person must be carrying the dominant gene for the particular 'trait'. We will call this dominant gene 'D'. A gene is represented on each one of a pair of chromosomes inherited from the mother and father. Therefore the affected person may also be carrying the recessive gene, 'd', for the condition. Such a person is termed a heterozygote, and the genetic make-up under consideration is summarised as 'Dd'. A 'Dd' parent must pass on either 'D' or 'd' to each of his or her children. 50% of the children of a heterozygote with an unaffected ('dd') partner may be expected to inherit the dominant gene. The expression of the dominant gene 'D' always overrides the expression of the recessive gene 'd'. Therefore, in the pattern of inheritance we are considering here, 50% of the children of an affected parent may be expected to be affected as well.

The affected person may be homozygote dominant. This means that the dominant gene form 'D' is represented on each member of the relevant pair of chromosomes. For the condition under review, the homozygote's genetic make-up is summarised as 'DD'. A 'DD' parent must pass on to his or her children the dominant gene 'D'. All the children of such a parent will be affected by the condition, regardless of the genetic make-up of the other parent. The genetic make-up of the spouse will decide whether the children are 'DD' or 'Dd'. The influence of this spouse on the amount of (for our interests) epilepsy expressed will be evident in the generation of grandchildren. The grandchildren may be genetically 'Dd' or 'DD' or 'dd' depending, in part, on the fortunes of partner selection.

Yet again it can be seen that the picture can be quite difficult to grasp but it is important to point out that an absolute answer to the probabilities of inheritance of epilepsy may not be possible in particular cases.

The above discussion has focused on a single type of inheritance pattern which assumes that the condition is inherited on a single gene, but in most conditions, probably including most types of epilepsy, there are a number of genes involved and the true situation cannot be so simply explained. What follows is not necessarily absolutely scientifically correct but it is offered to try to simplify what is really a very complex issue.

The best way to understand the complex picture is to assume that what is inherited is a threshold above which epileptic fits will occur. It has already been shown that almost everyone can have a fit, as was discussed with the condition known as deja vu. Thus everyone has a unique threshold for epileptic seizures. The obvious next question is to ask why everyone does not have a major convulsive seizure. The answer is that if people are sufficiently provoked they will have a convulsion. In other words, the reason that not everyone has experienced a convulsion is that not everyone has been stimulated beyond the threshold which protects against fits. Put yet another way, the person who has not had a convulsion has a threshold for convulsions that is considerably higher than that for the person with epilepsy.

If a person is given enough electric shock, or so much insulin that sugar levels fall very low, then he or she can be artificially provoked to have a fit. The difference is that the epileptic person needs less shock or insulin to have the same type of fit. This emphasises both the individual nature of the inheritance of epilepsy and the fact that the threshold for seizures is different for each person.

By now you may be really confused so, to simplify the situation, the position can be summarised by stating that **the inheritance of epilepsy depends on the seizure type, the syndrome type, the presence of associated illnesses and the addition of environmental factors** known to provoke fits in susceptible people. It can be seen that, like so many things in this book, each case should be considered on its individual merits but the simple answer is that epilepsy, or the tendency to recurrent seizures, is inherited but the nature of the inheritance and the expression of epilepsy to be anticipated in offspring requires careful deliberation in each case. Having said that, most doctors teach that in broad terms the risk of inheriting focal onset seizures, in the absence of other confounding factors, is very low and the risk of inheriting generalised forms of epilepsy is higher.

Other causes of epilepsy

It has already been established that **brain damage, brain tumour** (either primary tumour, derived from brain cells such as brain glial cells, or secondary deposits in the brain of metastasised tumour brought to the brain from other parts of the body such as the lungs), **electrolyte disturbance** (such as altered levels of sodium, potassium or calcium), **brain infections** (such as abscess or meningitis), **problems with sugar** (as found in diabetic patients), and **other bodily stresses** (such as urinary tract infections, asthma or migraine) can act as provocative factors in the person subject to fits. **Different causes are more common at different ages** and this will affect how the doctor investigates the patient in a particular age group.

In the elderly there are a number of common conditions, such as stroke or even Alzheimer's Disease, which are recognised to be associated with epilepsy. This is very logical because these conditions are either the cause or the result of brain damage and earlier material has already shown how brain damage can cause fits. This re-emphasises that conditions which affect the brain and have brain damage in their clinical picture can cause epilepsy, but it is also worth reiterating that prolonged epilepsy, as is found in status epilepticus, can itself cause brain damage.

When asked, it is important to realise that the question 'What causes epilepsy?' is really two questions rolled into one and, regrettably, it is easy to get away with only answering one of the two. The first answer is as given above, namely those medical conditions which are associated with fits in people with a lowered threshold to epileptic activity in the brain. The second question asks, 'What things will provoke fits in people who otherwise would not know that they may have epilepsy?'. Again, the answer to this question has already been given in part, both in the section dealing with EEG and also in earlier discussion in this chapter.

How to provoke a fit

As already stated, the EEG aims to map out abnormal brain activity and thus the conscientious doctor will ask the patient to do all those things known to enhance epileptic activity in the hope of provoking a fit during the recording of the EEG. These include: overbreathing (also called hyperventilation); opening and closing the eyes; sleep deprivation with associated fatigue and stress; drifting off to sleep; sleeping; waking up from sleep; looking at stroboscopic lights flashing at a variety of frequencies. In some people there are special triggers that can cause them to have fits and these can include everyday tasks such as eating, reading or writing.

Catamenial epilepsy

Epilepsy may be related to the **menstrual cycle and hormonal changes**, either at the time of ovulation or menstruation, which may result in the lowering of the body levels of anti-epileptic medications at these times. It has been argued that the brain can also be more sensitive to epileptic activity at these times in women who have not previously been on medication.

Alcohol and epilepsy

Alcohol can cause a person to have fits. This can happen in 3 different ways:

  (i) as a result of alcohol withdrawal
 (ii) as a direct result of alcohol toxicity which of itself has caused brain damage
(iii) as a result of head injury caused by being drunk, being therefore less careful and having an increase in accidents.

Epilepsy and drugs

As with a number of other drugs (and alcohol is not only a drug but a potential drug of addiction), the brain may become accustomed to the presence of the drug and stopping it suddenly can cause what are called **'withdrawal fits'**. Some of the drugs, other than alcohol, which are known to cause withdrawal fits are benzodiazepines (such as diazepam [Valium]) and barbiturates (such as phenobarbitone). It must be recognised that the anti-epileptic medications are also drugs and their sudden withdrawal can also cause a person to have a fit. This is the reason for the earlier comments in Chapter 5 which advised the observer to make sure that the person who is known to have epilepsy has taken his or her medications. Failure to take medications is a common cause of seizures.

There is another way in which drugs can cause fits. **Drugs can lower the threshold above which stimulation will cause fits to occur.** This is a little like the way alcohol causes fits due to direct toxicity. Some of the drugs known to affect the way the brain works, particularly the drugs used in psychiatry such as the antidepressants and the antipsychotics, have been reported to increase seizures and the cause is thought to be lowering of the threshold above which stimulation causes fits.

Chapter 7

If it is not epilepsy, what is it?

There are a number of conditions that can be confused with the diagnosis of epilepsy. It has been said that as many as one in four of the people referred to a specialist in epileptology with what was thought to be a definite diagnosis of epilepsy, does in fact not have epilepsy but has something else. Now is the moment to repeat the warning that it is far easier to apply the label of epilepsy than to remove it.

Psychological dependence on the diagnosis

While it seems strange to say it, some people become quite distressed when the diagnosis of epilepsy is removed and often may not accept that the diagnosis was inappropriately given in the first place. This may be part of the 'down side' to the use of video-telemetry. It has happened, on more than one occasion, that the video-EEG has proven that the patient does not have epilepsy and the only result has been that the patient changed doctors so that the diagnosis of epilepsy could be preserved, even if wrong! On occasions people need their illness to cope with life because it gives them an excuse when they find that they cannot do what is expected of them. It allows them to escape these embarrassing times. Often the doctor is ill-equipped to manage such situations because it is not usually part of medical training to learn to deal with patients who need to be sick and who are happier having a label which gives them a 'defence' for their own inadequacy.

Pseudoseizures

In pseudoseizures, now also referred to as non-epileptic seizures, the person has what is often thought to be a fit, but it
does not come from 'uncontrolled overactivity of part or all of
the brain' but rather from a psychological basis (meaning it is
caused by the emotions rather than by the effect of brain cells
overactive and beyond the person's control). Often the person
will not even be aware that they have such a psychological
force causing them to have a 'fit-look-alike' and the doctor has
to be very careful in dealing with this issue.

Sometimes it is very easy to tell the difference between
real and pseudo seizures, because what the person does in the
pseudoseizure could not happen unless it was under 'voluntary' control (even if such voluntary control is at the subconscious level). This is not always the case and often it is very
difficult to tell the difference between 'real' fits and these 'almost', non-epileptic, fits. This is one area in which video-
telemetry makes a real contribution because it allows both the
doctor and the patient to see just what is happening during an
event. It shows both the overt features of what the person does
in the so-called 'fit' as well as showing, inside the head, what
the brain is doing. It shows if there is epileptic brain activity
going on at the time of the 'fit' and permits the doctor to discuss
this with the patient. If there is no such epileptic activity it gives
a very good clue that what was seen was not a true 'fit' and
opens the door to clear and frank discussion with the patient or
relatives.

From a psychological point of view it is important to make
the distinction between real and pseudo (non-epileptic) seizures, because only after correct diagnosis can the doctor try to
treat the true cause of the problem or refer the patient to an
appropriate specialist, such as a psychiatrist. It is most important
to realise that the person may have no conscious awareness of
causing his or her own pseudoseizures and very important to
avoid treating this condition as one of 'wilful acting-out'. The
person may become quite hostile when confronted by the diagnosis, thinking that the doctor is making accusations of dishon-
esty and saying that he or she is doing it on purpose (which is
often not the case). This places the 'doctor–patient' relation-

ship at grave risk and it takes an experienced doctor to handle the situation properly, ensuring that everyone benefits from what is, in fact, the correct diagnosis and thus should help the patient's outcome.

As a rule of thumb, in pseudoseizures, the doctor needs to look for two things important in the management. These are (i) the identification of what is called the 'model' that shows the patient the behaviour upon which the 'fit-like' behaviour is based and (ii) an indication of the possible gain, or profit, for the patient as a result of having this type of pseudoseizure. (In other words the doctor needs to define both where the person learnt what to do in their pseudoseizures, and how these episodes help the person to get some desired benefit that would be denied them if they did not have pseudoseizures).

One of the most difficult problems in managing such patients is that often the person may be his or her own 'model', meaning that often the person who has pseudoseizures also has real epilepsy, and this can make treatment really difficult. For this person there is need to treat both the real epilepsy and the pseudoseizures and there is need to educate the patient about the difference between the two.

The management of pseudoseizures can be a very complex problem and will not be discussed in great detail as this book is directed specifically towards the person with epilepsy rather than those with other conditions. It is hoped that the information given will allow you to better understand some of the difficulties involved in telling the differences between real and pseudoseizures, and will encourage further reading.

Syncope or faints

Perhaps the most common condition to be confused with epilepsy is the 'simple faint', which is called **syncope or syncopal attack** in 'medical talk'. A faint is usually a short lived thing in which the person may feel light-headed before the episode and then lose consciousness for a very short period of time. **One of the confusing things in a syncopal attack is that the person may have a very short period of time when they get insufficient blood to their brain and in that time they can shake in a way that looks like a fit.** This resemblance is called 'epileptiform' and highlights the difficulty that may be experienced in the establishment of a proper diagnosis.

After the faint the person rapidly returns to normal, something that often distinguishes it from a fit which is usually followed by a short period when the person is confused and does not know where they are or what happened. The faint may be caused by a number of conditions, such as: irregular heart rate; excessive heat; excessive stimulation of the vagal nerve, which causes such things as dilatation of the blood vessels as well as rapid heart rate and lowering of blood pressure and is called a **vaso-vagal episode**.

Need for cardiological assessment

In this situation the person needs to be fully investigated and often the full range of tests done for the person with epilepsy will be needed for this type of patient. This is especially so if the history is not absolutely clear. It is often important to order heart investigations, such as holter monitor ECG, in which the patient carries a heart monitor with them for a long period, often a full 24-hour day; that is then read by an experienced cardiologist to look for heart irregularities. Other heart tests such as echo-cardiograph may be needed. This uses sound waves to map out what the heart looks like so that the doctor can see if there are any blood clots or other abnormalities in the heart. There are a number of ways now of doing echo-cardiographs, such as doing the test through the skin, on the chest wall, or actually placing the device down the food pipe (the oesophagus) and sending the waves to the heart from within the body. The decision as to which technique to use depends on the skill of the heart doctor, the availability of equipment and exactly why the test is being done. Again, further discussion of this point is beyond the scope of this book.

Breath-holding attacks and night terrors

In children, **breath-holding attacks** and **night terrors** are two conditions that are often confused with epilepsy. A good history is often all that is required to tell the difference but in some cases it can also be very difficult to distinguish between these events and genuine epilepsy. In breath-holding attacks there is often a situation, before the onset of the episode, which indicates that the child is experiencing frustration or anger or even shock which is expressed by the breath-holding episode. A good history is the most important tool in this case. Night terrors often happen shortly after the child has gone to bed, often after a very busy day, and have the child in a state of absolute fear, often crying or screaming, for no obvious reason; the parent has a great deal of trouble pacifying the frightened child and getting him or her to go back to bed.

Both night terrors and breath-holding attacks are very frightening, especially for the parents, and it is important to put their minds at ease so that they can come to terms with the problem. Sometimes it is necessary to investigate the child, both to be certain that the diagnosis is correct, as well as to be able to reassure the parents that the diagnosis is correct, based on the test results which can be shown to them! Video-EEG is very valuable in this context and often helps the doctor to make the correct diagnosis.

Hyperventilation

Hyperventilation (overbreathing) may cause light-headedness and a tingling sensation throughout the body. It may cause the person to collapse, hands and face muscles may become very tight and he or she may shake. The person may have true **vertigo** as a result of the hyperventilation. Vertigo is an unreal sensation that the room is spinning or moving when it is not. It can occur as part of a complex partial seizure but usually it has nothing to do with epilepsy and is yet another condition which can be confused with epilepsy. Again it may be difficult to tell the difference between epilepsy and hyperventilation in some patients who have a confusing history and there may be need to fully investigate the patient before being confident about this diagnosis.

To make it even more difficult, it has already been shown that hyperventilation can be used to bring on a fit while an EEG is being undertaken, and it must be remembered that even those with diagnosed epilepsy can have episodes of self-induced hyperventilation if they are anxious people.

Myoclonic jerks that are not epileptic

Patients often come to the doctor because of strange movements experienced, usually, in bed just before going to sleep. These may be described as a jumping sensation, or a feeling as if about to fall off a cliff. For the patient, these are very real and can be quite disturbing. They are called **'hypnagogic myoclonus'** and should not be confused with epilepsy. They usually do not require further investigation. It is important to realise that these are very common and that most people have experienced them at some time in their life. The person who comes to the doctor with a whole range of strange, and not so strange, movement symptoms may be scared that he or she has epilepsy when this is not so. This is not to say that this person may not have some other form of significant neurological disorder that requires attention.

Sleep disorders

Recently there has been a resurgence of interest in sleep disorders and it has been shown that a significant number of people thought to have epilepsy, due to the reporting of strange episodes during the day, do not have epilepsy but have conditions such as sleep apnoea (stopping breathing during sleep). This can cause excessive tiredness due to lack of oxygen to the brain throughout the night, and as a result the person may 'drift off' in the day. Without evidence to the contrary it may be assumed that these episodes represent absences or complex partial seizures.

The test to be undertaken is an all-night diagnostic polysomnographic sleep study (a sophisticated test which involves applying numerous electrodes to the patient to measure brain-waves, heart rate, breathing, oxygen in the blood, movement and snoring, and observing the patient overnight in a specialised sleep laboratory, under the supervision of a trained sleep technician who is experienced in sleep medicine). This test should be considered in all patients who have early onset snoring during a routine or sleep deprived EEG. It should be considered in all obese patients who present with a suspicious history which suggests hypersomnolence (excessive sleepiness) or who are known to be 'heavy snorers'. If there is doubt about the diagnosis then the sleeping partner should be interviewed and asked about the patient's snoring habits and if he or she sits up at night, woken from sleep, gasping for air.

Other sleep disorders include some of the so-called parasomnias (abnormal behaviours which accompany sleep). These include sleep-walking (also called somnambulism), some of the movement disorders associated with sleep such as the sleep dystonias (further discussion of which is beyond the scope of this book) and restless leg syndrome (also called Periodic Leg [or Limb] Movement in Sleep, PLMS). Upper airway resistance syndrome (UARS), which causes breathing problems due to a difficulty getting air into the lungs, may also affect sleep and cause disturbed sleep patterns resulting in excessive fatigue.

It should not be ignored that sleep disorders can also impact upon real epilepsy by causing sleep deprivation which has already been identified as a potent cause for provoking fits in susceptible people. It follows that a proper consideration of possible sleep disorders should be a part of the evaluation of all patients referred with a potential diagnosis of epilepsy.

Other epilepsy look-alikes

Some of the other conditions that deserve a mention in a chapter dealing with 'epilepsy look-alikes' include: Gilles de la Tourette syndrome; cataplexy; schizophrenia and other psychiatric disorders.

Gilles de la Tourette is a condition associated with tics (unusual brief movements of the muscles) and grunts, sniffing, snorting, the tendency to repeat what was just said (like an echo) and a compulsive urge to swear and use bad language. Because of the movements it is sometimes called epilepsy but it should not be considered part of the epilepsies.

Cataplexy is associated with narcolepsy. A person has a cataplectic episode when he or she collapses at times of emotional excitement, such as when jokes are told or he or she has an upset. Because of the fall, the episode may be confused with an epileptic seizure.

Schizophrenia is associated with hallucinations and sometimes these are confused with overactivity of the brain as is seen in epilepsy. Psychiatrists have devised a classification system, referred to as the DSM IVR, which categorises 'mental' or psychiatric sicknesses. The problem with schizophrenia is that, depending upon the literature reviewed, between 5 and 80% of sufferers may have an abnormal EEG and evidence to suggest either frontal or temporal lobe involvement. As with epilepsy, schizophrenia is now divided into a variety of conditions called schizophrenia and schizophreniform conditions. Further discussion of schizophrenia is beyond the scope of this book. Often the strange behaviour seen in psychiatric disorders is confused with automatisms (automatic behaviour seen in complex partial seizures), and sometimes the only way to really differentiate between the two categories of conditions is to have video-telemetry at the time of such behaviour.

Again the complexity that is epileptology has been emphasised and it should be restated that not everything that collapses and shakes is epileptic; there are many conditions that cause involuntary movements or in which the person may seem to be distracted and yet the person does not have epilepsy. The doctor needs to exclude conditions that can be confused with epilepsy before that diagnosis is applied. The first job of the doctor who sees a patient labelled as epileptic is to make sure that the diagnosis has been given correctly. It cannot be stated too often that the diagnosis of epilepsy is not a benign diagnosis.

The need for a positive diagnosis

The diagnosis of epilepsy carries with it many limitations on the person's ability to enjoy life to the full. The doctor has to be 100% certain that the diagnosis has been correctly applied. This chapter has highlighted just some of the areas in which confusion may arise but it is important to emphasise that this is not offered as an absolutely complete list of confounding diagnoses; you are encouraged to read further and to question constantly what has happened thus far in the management if there is any doubt.

Keep in mind the cautionary saying, 'One does not buy one's pool from the first person who quotes for its construction!'. The same advice applies to the delivery of medical care and if there is doubt then you should start asking questions and, if the answers are not satisfactory, never be afraid to seek a second opinion.

The problem with seeking a second opinion is that there is no guarantee that the second opinion is correct just because it differs from the first opinion. It is always wise to seek the second opinion in an open fashion so that the first doctor knows that it is being sought. This allows the first doctor the right of reply and gives the patient some degree of protection against a wrong second opinion. The patient needs to be satisfied that the final decision as to whom to trust is arrived at by a sensible and correct approach, and giving the first doctor the right of reply goes a long way to achieving this.

Chapter 8

How is epilepsy treated?

The next step in the management of the patient who has epilepsy depends on the diagnosis that has been made and the cause that may have been found. **If the condition diagnosed and the cause are treatable then that should dictate the focus of future attention.** This may seem a self-explanatory and unnecessary statement but is best justified by the following example.

Treat the cause of the seizures before treating the epilepsy!

It seems wrong to place an alcoholic on medication to treat epilepsy if the diagnosis is that of alcoholism. The focus of attention should be directed towards treatment of the alcoholism and helping the person to stop drinking alcohol and to overcome dependence on an addictive substance. There are two reasons for this approach, the first of which is that it is the alcoholism that is the primary problem and proper care should always be aimed at correcting the basic illness. The second reason is that alcoholics are notoriously poor at compliance with prescribed treatment, so that, even if the doctor prescribes anti-epileptic medication, there is a significant risk that the alcoholic patient will not take the medication according to the doctor's instructions.

Similarly, if the person has had seizures because of a brain lesion, then the right approach is to make sure that one knows what the brain abnormality is and then to treat that pathology in the correct way. If the person has a tumour then it should be treated correctly, by removal, radiotherapy, or whatever the cancer doctors suggest, before the person is given years of anti-epileptic medicines which will not address the primary problem. However, even if the tumour is removed, there may still be need for on-going use of anti-epileptic medication to protect the patient against seizures which may result from abnormalities that persist within the brain.

If there is an abscess it should be treated as such, rather than the person being labelled epileptic and the primary illness ignored. Infections need antibiotics. Abnormal blood vessels (such as arterio-venous malformations) need to be treated by either neurosurgeons or very specialised radiologists so as to either remove the abnormal collection of vessels or block the abnormal blood vessels, so protecting the patient against future bleeds and the very predictable recurrence of seizures.

The first-things-first approach should not deny the person access to the correct anti-epileptic medicines if these are required to give the person protection against further fits. What it must do is make sure that the person has the best treatment available for the primary cause of the fits. In some cases, even after it has been clearly established that there is a primary cause for the epilepsy, and that cause has been correctly treated (with surgery, or whatever other forms of treatment are indicated), it may still be necessary for the person to be on anti-epileptic treatment for a short period. This may be only for about six months while everything settles down. However it is not always so simple and some people will need to be on anti-epileptic medication for life, even after correct management of the primary condition. As always, **each case must be considered on its merits and be treated as a unique situation**.

Having treated the cause, now treat the epilepsy!

Once the primary cause for the epilepsy has been addressed and correctly treated then the focus of treatment can be directed specifically at the treatment of the fits. While acknowledging the unique nature of each case, there are some basic guidelines that can be stated to help the doctor in the decision-making process and ensure the optimal choice of medicine.

As set out earlier, the choice of medication is determined by the type of fit and perhaps the type of epilepsy. Each doctor will have his or her own favoured choice of medicine for each seizure type and what follows reflects my choice and preferences but need not reflect the choice of any other doctor. Having said that, I also want to say that the choices set out in the following passages have not been developed without considerable experience in the area of epileptology. They are not merely arbitrary decisions, but reflect my years of practice in treating people with epilepsy. In the following sections which look at drug treatment of epilepsy, I will give my personal views as to the relative place of the different drugs.

For the purposes of this book I have used generic names (such as valproate or ethosuximide), rather than trade names. But, recognising that each drug has both a generic name, one that is universally accepted, and a trade name or names, which may be specific to each country in which the drug is used, generic and trade names will be provided together at least once, to allow you to identify the medicine about which I am writing.

The long-established anti-epileptic medications

The history of the modern era of epilepsy treatment dates back to the mid 18th century with a report of the use of **bromides**. These are no longer widely used, so I won't discuss them here. However, I know of one very senior epileptologist who still uses bromides in selected cases.

The next anti-epileptic medication to be reported was the barbiturate, **phenobarbitone**, in 1912, and while I do not prescribe phenobarbitone I do prescribe **primidone** on an occasional basis as a third or fourth line agent. Primidone is metabolised in the body to phenobarbitone, and both primidone and phenobarbitone have anti-epileptic properties. Phenobarbitone is useful in the treatment of most forms of epilepsy but particularly generalised seizures, especially myoclonic seizure, when other agents fail.

Phenobarbitone is said to work on controlling seizures in a

variety of ways. These may include limiting the spread of seizure activity, elevating the seizure threshold, and suppressing
the release of excitatory neurotransmitters, such as glutamate
and aspartate. It acts on the sodium/potassium movement in and
out of the brain cells.

Phenobarbitone causes problems with mental activity, such
as thinking, concentration and memory, and with emotions. It
makes people tired and, especially in children it is noted to
make them very moody. It has a long half-life of about 3 days,
and it takes a long time to reach steady state (the level at which
its blood level remains relatively static between doses). It stimulates production of liver enzymes and consequently the blood
levels of other anti-epileptic medications usually fall, diminishing their effects.

There are a number of medications currently available, such
as methylphenobarbitone (Prominal) and primidone (Mysoline),
which are metabolised to phenobarbitone in the body and
which work as phenobarbitone. Primidone may have an anti-
epileptic role even before it is metabolised to phenobarbitone.
I use primidone in preference to phenobarbitone because of
this fact. The only time I do use phenobarbitone itself is for the
treatment of status epilepticus which has failed to respond to
other agents, because it is one of the few anti-epileptic agents
that can be administered by intramuscular injection and has a
fairly predictable absorption rate. The blood level can be measured and compared with the reported therapeutic range. The
risk with phenobarbitone, in status epilepticus, is respiratory
depression and this risk needs to be emphasised to the supervising staff.

Phenytoin was the next anti-epileptic agent to be reported; in
1938 its properties were documented by Merritt and Putnam,
whose names live on in scientific meetings sponsored in their
honour around the world. Phenytoin was the first agent to be
proven effective in epilepsy experimentation in animals before it
was used in people. It has the most successful history of any of
the anti-epileptic medications in that it is still used as a first line
medication by many doctors. I no longer use it as first choice
because of its many side effects, including acne, hirsutism (hairiness), cognitive (intellectual function) impairment, gingivitis (inflammation of the gums) and a whole host of other unwanted

effects. Phenytoin has a difficult metabolism of the type known as saturation metabolism. The body approaches limitations to its ability to process phenytoin; consequently, at high dose which may change from one patient to another, a tiny increase in dosage can cause a great change in the blood levels of phenytoin and a surge in adverse effects.

Phenytoin is said to act by stopping the spread of seizure activity and suppressing sustained high-frequency repetitive firing of neurones in the excited state.

The role of phenytoin, in my hands, is as second, or third, line therapy in partial seizures, including simple partial, complex partial and secondarily generalised tonic/clonic seizures. It is ineffective in absence fits and is not very useful in the other generalised seizures. It, too, has a long half-life, although much shorter than the barbiturates, of up to $1\frac{1}{2}$ days and so it takes considerable time to reach steady-state. For this reason there is little point checking blood levels in under 2 weeks. Because of its long half-life many doctors prescribe it on a once a day regimen, but I do not do so because I have found that patients do not always do as the doctor prescribes and may miss a dose, which means that there could easily be 2 days between doses. I therefore prescribe it on a twice daily regimen, which means that if the patient misses a dose then he or she will still get half the dose or can catch up and take the full daily dose in one go on realising what has happened.

Phenytoin is metabolised in the liver and in general lowers the level of other anti-epileptic medications when given in polypharmacy.

Phenytoin can be given by intravenous injection for status epilepticus but it must be remembered that it is cardiac active and in years gone by was used to correct irregularities in heart rhythms (it prolongs the conduction at the atrio-venticular node). Overseas, the agent phosphenytoin is available, which is easier to give either intravenously or intramuscularly, and is effective for status epilepticus.

Ethosuximide was introduced to clinical practice in 1958 and its sole role in the treatment of epilepsy is as first or second line therapy for the treatment of primarily generalised absence seizures. Its short coming is that it may increase the tendency for major generalised convulsive seizures and hence it is not a first line agent in my adult practice. In young children it is often chosen by paediatricians because it is much less likely to interfere with liver function than is valproate.

Carbamazepine was first written up in 1963 for use in trigeminal neuralgia, and in the same year for treatment of epilepsy. It has replaced phenytoin as my first choice in the treatment of partial seizures and I sometimes add it to treatments begun with other anti-epileptic medications in some of the generalised epilepsies, such as those with primarily generalised tonic/clonic seizures. Compared to phenytoin, it is much easier to predict the blood level of drug that will result from dosing with carbamazapine. Its side effect profile is less intrusive than that of phenytoin especially with regard to the cosmetic side effects which are often intolerable to young adolescents who have enough to cope with in the face of having epilepsy at this difficult time in their lives.

Carbamazepine evolved during the development of the anti-depressant imipramine, and because of similarity in structure carbamazepine, also, has been gaining favour as a psychotropic agent and as an analgesic in situations of neuralgias. It is also metabolised in the liver and is known to stimulate production of the liver enzymes controlling its own metabolism. Consequently, blood levels of carbamazepine fall after about 4 weeks usage. It is my practice, therefore, to delay use of blood level monitoring till 6 weeks after introduction of carbamazepine by which stage there should be stable levels.

There are standard tablets and controlled release formulations of carbamazepine. It also comes in a syrup, which is used for children, and I have also used the syrup formulation given per rectum as an enema in patients who could not be given oral medications for whatever reasons. There is no injectable preparation of carbamazepine available in Australia. Many practitioners prescribe three times a day dosing with carbamazepine because its half-life is approximately $^{1}/_{3}$ to 1 day (shorter than the half-life of either phenytoin or the barbiturates). I do not use three times a day dosage because it has been my experience that the midday dosage is often not taken and hence the compliance is not adequate. The controlled release tablets are designed to reinforce the approach of twice daily dosage but the family doctor needs to be warned that I have had significant problems changing from the standard preparation to the controlled release formulation; there is not a direct bioequivalence of dosages and it cannot be assumed that 400mg CR (controlled release) carbamazepine is equivalent to 400mg of the standard preparation. While the experts claim 20% reduction in bioequivalence I have found the change to be less predictable than that and caution must be exercised when changing from one formulation to the other.

Because of the liver metabolism there is usually a lowering of the level of other medications with the addition of carbamazepine to treatment. The one situation which is a little different is the combined use of phenytoin and carbamazepine. The patient is usually on phenytoin when referred to me. The reason for referral is often that phenytoin is not effective enough, and so I add carbamazepine to the treatment. However, the patient may report toxicity and blame the carbamazepine, claiming an allergy to it. This is usually not the case. What has happened is that the addition of carbamazepine has resulted in the elevation of the phenytoin levels and the patient may well be phenytoin toxic due to the polypharmacy combination. This is when blood level monitoring has particular value in determining the true offending agent.

Like the other anti-epileptic medications already described, carbamazepine interacts with some non-epileptic agents, such as the oral contraceptive pill, and may lower the effectiveness of the pill. The one interaction that should be highlighted is the interaction with erythromycin because this antibiotic is often used in patients who are allergic to penicillin and these patients are concerned about reactions to medications. Erythromycin has the potential to significantly increase the level of carbamazepine and thus can cause carbamazepine toxicity which this type of patient may interpret as an allergic reaction. The patient should be warned of the potential interaction, and, blood level monitoring is invaluable if assessment is needed.

The side effect profile of carbamazepine is not so different, with regard to higher centre function and central nervous system effects, when compared with other anti-epileptic medications, such as phenytoin. However, carbamazepine seems more likely to cause eye movement effects and skin rashes. (It also causes lowering of the level of electrolytes, such as sodium and chloride [which respond to fluid restriction] and affects the blood picture with lowering of the white cell count and increased potential for agranulocytosis.)

1963 was also the year that **valproate** was first recognised as an anti-epileptic medication. Prior to that time it had been used as the solvent in drug trials and it was the Belgian couple Meunier and Meunier who suggested its role as an active compound in the treatment of epilepsy. Since its introduction it has been recognised as the anti-epileptic agent with the widest range of effectiveness, and is the principal medication of choice in the treatment of primarily generalised seizures; it is also effective to about the same extent as carbamazepine in partial seizures. It has been said that if there is any doubt about the classification of a seizure then valproate is the agent of choice.

The anti-epileptic effect of valproate was initially thought to come exclusively from its action in enhancing the activity of the inhibitory neurotransmitter GABA. More recently it has been suggested that valproate may have a range of activities, such as affecting calcium currents, which explain its wide ranging effectiveness.

Valproate is available as a 100 mg uncoated tablet and as 200 mg and 500 mg enteric coated tablets, and as a liquid to be taken by mouth. It must be remembered that valproate is easily soluble in water and so the uncoated tablet is very susceptible to exposure to everyday humidity and should not be taken out of the wrapper until about to be taken, the exposed tablet should not be kept in a dosing container, as is sometimes the practice when treatment is prepared well in advance.

The half-life of valproate is reported to be between $^1/_3$ and $^1/_2$ a day, but I still use a twice daily regimen of therapy, for the same reasons I gave earlier. Many clinicians dispute the use of blood level monitoring in valproate treatment, but I rely heavily on such monitoring because I use higher dosages of valproate than almost any of my colleagues; I do so with strict monitoring of both total drug and free drug blood levels, and the biochemical and full blood picture profiles, recognising that valproate has a notorious reputation for liver toxicity, and potential fatality, especially in the young, and it also lowers blood parameters, especially the platelets. (The meaning of 'total' and 'free' drug levels is discussed a little later in this chapter in a section on blood level monitoring.)

More recently, valproate has been named as a possible cause of polycystic ovaries, and it is well known to be associated with obesity, thought to relate to an appetite stimulation effect. Another problem with valproate is that it has been shown to be associated with increased risk of spina bifida in the unborn infant; use of folic acid in the pregnancy does offer some protection against this.

Valproate is the medicine of choice in treating situation related epilepsy, such as photoconvulsive seizures. In Australia the injectable formulation is not yet available, but rectal administration of the oral syrup has proven effective in situations in which the patient could not take oral agents, and in the case of status epilepticus.

Of the benzodiazepines, **clonazepam**, used as an anti-epileptic agent since 1975, and, more recently, **clobazam**, recognised as an anti-epileptic medication since 1978, are the most popular members. I am not a great supporter of the use of benzodiazepines in the long-term treatment of epilepsy because of problems with tolerance (requiring increasingly larger doses of the agent for the same effect) and the side effect profile of fatigue and irritability and mood swings. They do have their devotees, particularly for the treatment of the generalised epilepsies, but in my hands their major contribution is in the treatment of situation related epilepsies. If it is known that certain situations provoke seizures, such as an unwelcome visit or menstruation or a stressful sporting trial or school examination, I may use them for short periods, with good effect. I will sometimes use **lorazepam** as a very short acting benzodiazepine in this situation, if I feel a single dose may be all that is required before a football match or a once-off interview, but I will get the patient to try the medication on a day, when excessive sedation or irritability will be no problem. Only if a patient tolerates the medication will I then use it as 'pulse' therapy in provocative situations.

Other benzodiazepines are of some use in the treatment of epilepsy. **Diazepam** is used both as a tranquilliser and by injection for status epilepticus; it should not be given intramuscularly, however, because of unreliable absorption. Rectal administration is used in emergencies. **Midazolam** is of use as a water soluble intramuscular injection for the treatment of status epilepticus. It is also reported to be given by nasal application.

Nitrazepam and **temazepam** are useful as hypnotics in patients who are sleep deprived and in whom it is advisable to assist sleep to ensure seizure control. Anxiolytics such as **oxazepam** have some role to play but in these situations I favour clobazam, which I have found to be better tolerated than clonazepam; it causes less side effects.

The exciting new anti-epileptic medicines

It is a very exciting time to be working in the care of those with epilepsy because there are a whole range of new anti-epileptic medicines available and being developed. However, it is only after 'coal face' use of the drugs, in routine clinical practice, that the real place and use of each agent emerges. My remarks here are not intended as a criticism of the governmental assessment process but reflect changes in understanding of their functions that have emerged with the use of some of the newer medications since they were registered for general use within the community.

In the Australian health care system, medications are assessed by the Drug Safety and Evaluation branch of Therapeutic Goods Administration following application by the drug companies and on information supplied, in a set format, by them. Recommendations are passed on to the independent Australian Drug Evaluation Committee (ADEC) which issues approvals for specific indications. Registration follows approval. It is a lengthy process!

I have recently surveyed my colleagues to see how my opinions on the new drugs are matched by their practice and it was really quite revealing to see how the newer medicines have already attracted a considerable degree of acceptance. There is already quite a divergence between approved indications for these newer agents and their actual application to patient care in routine clinical practice. This is most apparent with lamotrigine which has recently been registered in many countries, including Australia, as 'add-on' therapy for refractory partial seizures. One of the respondents of my survey indicated that lamotrigine should be considered as a first line treatment in generalised seizures even though it is not registered in Australia for this indication.

It is with this in mind that I offer my personal views to help you look into the future and get a feel for the newer medicines, some of which are only available from special centres with a particular interest in epileptology.

These newer agents include vigabatrin (Sabril), lamotrigine (Lamictal), gabapentin (Neurontin), tiagabine (Gabatril), topiramate (Topamax), felbamate (Taloxa), plus remacemide, stiripentol, dezinamide, zonisamide, rufinamide. There are a number of medicines, such as ucb L059, that have not yet been given names, and are still referred to by company development numbers. Some companies have identified even newer agents that look as though they may be useful in the management of epilepsy but animal studies on these medicines have not been completed and to date they have not been given to people, or given to so few people that further discussion is inappropriate. It follows that there is good reason for epileptics to be optimistic but it is fair to say that epileptologists still feel that the 'magic bullet' has not yet surfaced and we wait with expectation.

Of the agents listed above, **felbamate** has recently received a severe blow because the risk of developing aplastic anaemia from its use has been found to be of the order of 1/10 000. This seems an unacceptable risk for many people and definitely so for those with newly diagnosed epilepsy because other approved medicines have a far lower, though still present, risk of this unwanted effect. This would seem to make the use of felbamate, in this context, unacceptable. There are also reports of liver problems with this medicine, yet it is still approved for marketing in the USA.

Zonisamide is another of the new agents tested in Australia, as was felbamate, and in many other countries. While it proved to be an effective anti-epileptic medicine, it caused what was considered an unacceptable increase in the risk of kidney stones (according to the company which was sponsoring the trials) and thus the trials were stopped in most countries. Zonisamide was developed in Japan and is still used in that country. There is talk that the drug may be tested again in the rest of the world but the picture is not clear.

Topiramate is currently being tested in Australia and has recently been registered for sale and launched in Australia in August 1997. There are questions of kidney stone formation being associated with the use of this medicine but the company which has developed this drug feels that the risks are not high enough to justify stopping the development of the agent. Of those who have had kidney stones while on this medicine, about 75% elected to continue to take the drug. It must be remembered that the numbers involved are very small but the experience with this trial has been taken to suggest that the patients were happy with what they had gained from taking topiramate. It is still too early to know what the future holds with this medicine. As is the problem with scientific trials of anti-epileptic medications, the indications and dosages used represent somewhat of a gamble, and with topiramate there is a suggestion that the dosage trialed was too high, thereby causing some misconceptions about appropriate use in clinical practice.

Another of the new generation of anti-epileptic drugs, developed in Europe, is **oxcarbazepine (Trileptil)**. This medicine was a by-product of the development of carbamazepine but is said to have far fewer brain side effects and is preferred to carbamazepine in parts of Scandinavia where it was trialed for more than 10 years. There has been a resurgence of interest in this drug with new trials undertaken in Australia. The company responsible for its development has gone through a merger and it will take a little time for the dust to settle before the new management's ethos and its intentions regarding this medicine become clear. It is quite difficult to get oxcarbazepine for routine use; approach to the Special Access Scheme section of the Pharmaceutical Benefits Scheme will sometimes result in approval for compassionate use in selected patients. I do have patients on it and it seems a very effective medication, at least as effective as carbamazepine. My personal experience has been that some of the claims, particularly those relating to the low cross-sensitivity for skin rash, are a little over-enthusiastic but, this aside, I am impressed with its improved effect on fatigue and unwanted cognitive effects.

Tiagabine has been tested in Australia and has now been registered for use in Europe. As with many of the new anti-epileptic medications, its final role in the overall management of epilepsy remains to be defined. There is a suggestion that it may have a special role in the treatment of the elderly and in the management of Simple Partial Seizures but this is still based on anecdotal (non-scientific experience) reports and awaits further, scientific, confirmation.

Vigabatrin, lamotrigine and **gabapentin** have all been registered for sale in Australia for some years now and are rapidly being introduced into the care of patients with epilepsy who have failed to respond to older anti-epileptic medicines. All of these drugs are currently undergoing, or have undergone, trials to assess if they can be given as monotherapy to patients newly diagnosed with epilepsy, but it is still too early to be dogmatic. It would seem that all three will jump this hurdle eventually, but for now they are primarily used as 'add-on' treatments and economic factors may preclude their acceptability as front-line agents for newly diagnosed patients.

It is worth mentioning that the newer agents were all first tested in patients with focal epilepsy because it is easier to find such patients who have had difficult-to-manage epilepsy and so are willing to be part of clinical trials. Many of these new drugs have now been developed to the point where companies are testing them in newly diagnosed epileptics. The next real challenge will be to decide which of these medicines will be the best agent and in what circumstances the benefits will be maximised.

Treatment of absence seizures

Absence fits are best treated with either sodium valproate (Epilim) or ethosuximide (Zarontin). I favour valproate for absence fits because it has a wider range of efficacy as it covers all generalised epilepsies, and also gives reasonable benefit in treating focal epilepsies. On the other hand, ethosuximide is ineffective in treating tonic/clonic convulsive seizures and may even increase the risk of experiencing these. Paediatricians often favour ethosuximide because there is a risk of liver problems in children under the age of 2 who are exposed to valproate.

Treatment of other generalised epilepsies

The agent of choice for generalised epilepsies, at this point in time, is **sodium valproate**, although some of the other agents also have a role to play. Benzodiazepines, such as **clonazepam**

(Rivotril) or **clobazam (Frisium)**, have a role in the treatment of generalised epilepsies, such as absences, myoclonic fits and convulsive seizures.

A problem with clobazam is that it has not undergone extensive trialling to prove its value in the treatment of epilepsy and the government has only officially recognised its value in the treatment of anxiety states. This has attracted much criticism from many epileptologists and a direct appeal from the drugs advisory committee of the Epilepsy Society of Australia, but this has failed to change the current Australian position. Thus the long term safety of clobazam has not been proved which means that the government cannot recommend its prolonged use for epileptics. As a result of this, clobazam is not listed as a benefit on the Pharmaceutical Benefits Scheme and is very expensive if used on a long term basis in the amounts recommended by epileptologists.

All the members of the **benzodiazepine family of drugs** have an effect in the treatment of epilepsy. These drugs include **nitrazepam (Mogadon), oxazepam (Serepax), lorazepam (Ativan)** and a wide variety of anxiolytic medicines which are usually used as tranquillisers. Like clobazam, none of these agents have been proven to be safe, in formal clinical trials, for the long term use that is required in epilepsy. However, they have been used in this way for many years and epileptologists are satisfied that in some patients the use of these drugs is effective and highly recommended.

The problem with the benzodiazepines is that the patient may develop what is called 'tolerance' to the drugs, which means that the person needs more and more of the same medicine to get the effect that they once had on a lower dose. Put another way, the body becomes used to the drug and thus needs more of it to do the same job.

Barbiturates (including **primidone [Mysoline], methylphenobarbitone [Prominal]** and **phenobarbitone [phenobarb]**) also have a role in the treatment of generalised epilepsies. A common problem with both benzodiazepines and barbiturates is that if the agent is stopped suddenly then the patient is at considerable risk of withdrawal fits (as were described in Chapter 6).

Of the newer agents that are either being developed, or

which have been developed and registered for sale, **lamotrigine and gabapentin seem to have a role in the management of the generalised epilepsies although the appraisal of the trial of gabapentin in generalised epilepsy has not been as encouraging as I feel it should have been. The results of controlled trials are not to hand with lamotrigine but prepublished information and anecdotal reports fully endorse its use in this type of seizure disorder.** Tiagabine is also being appraised for use in Primarily Generalised Epilepsy but it is too early to have any useful data.

This highlights the gulf that sometimes appears between clinical medicine and scientific research, hence the rider stating that what appears in this book is based on my clinical judgment rather than on purely scientific publication. It is important, however, to inform you when there is discrepancy between the two. **Lamotrigine has been reported to be effective for Lennox Gastaut Syndrome but again no controlled trials have yet been reported.**

Felbamate was reported to be effective in the treatment of Lennox Gastaut Syndrome and thus it is to be expected that felbamate would have a role to play in the treatment of generalised epilepsies, if it were to complete the developmental process, something that now seems unlikely.

None of these new agents has been registered for use specifically in patients with generalised epilepsies. This situation merely reflects a failure of drug trials to pose the questions and supply the answers necessary before the government will approve use of these agents within this context, and emphasises the points raised above with regard to clinical experience. **Lack of specific approval does not prevent the doctor's use of these drugs in these situations and it may be wise, for the informed patient to ask the doctor to indicate if the drug has been approved for the use for which the doctor has prescribed it.**

The patient should not be embarrassed to question why the doctor has chosen to use a particular drug for that patient's epilepsy. The patient has every right to know what agent is being used and why it was chosen. The patient also has the right to know if the medicine was approved to be used in the way the doctor has elected to use it and, if not, why not. **Patients should not give up their human rights as part of their doctor/patient relationship and should ask questions.**

Treatment of reflex epilepsies

In the reflex epilepsies, such as photoconvulsive epilepsy, the drug of choice is valproate. Other agents which might have a role to play in the reflex epilepsies are lamotrigine and tiagabine. Preclinical experimental work in animals showed their efficacy in the epilepsy of photosensitivity.

Treatment of partial seizures/focal epilepsy

Partial seizures, as found in the focal epilepsies, are best treated with carbamazepine (Tegretol), valproate or phenytoin (Dilantin), probably in that order. Of the newer generation of anti-epileptic agents, vigabatrin, lamotrigine, gabapentin, tiagabine and probably remacemide and topiramate will all have a role to play.

Choice of medicine and dosage

You will note that actual dosages of medicines have not been discussed and the reason is because these are dependent upon each individual case. The doctor will usually build up the amount of the drug used in small incremental doses. The basic rule is that the patient should not be on either one more, nor one less, tablet than is needed to control the fits. The doctor will start with the smallest amount of the drug that he or she feels should control the epilepsy.

The choice of medicine is determined by the broad guidelines as set out above but the best use of these agents is set by the experience and preference of the doctor. The doctor decides how much medicine is right for a patient by giving sufficient medicine to stop the fits, or by giving the medicine in increasing amounts until the patient has side effects which mean he or she cannot tolerate a higher dose of the drug.

The use of drug level monitoring

Some people say that a drug should be given to patients who are still fitting to a dosage that produces at least a blood level of the medicine that is at, or just above, the upper end of **the therapeutic window**. The therapeutic window is the range of blood levels reported to show the amount of the drug, which controls the epilepsy, without side effect, in a population sample. Not all the drugs have an accepted therapeutic range which is believed to reflect the clinical efficacy of the medicine in the fashion described above. (An example of this is the benzodiazepine family of drugs.)

At times there is a debate as to what drug levels should be measured, assuming that levels should be measured at all. In some cases the drug has an active metabolite and there is also debate as to whether one should measure the level of such a metabolite. Carbamazepine provides an example of this issue. One can measure the **total drug level** of carbamazepine in the blood (that is the amount that is bound to the proteins that are in the blood plus the amount that is free within the blood and hence not protein-bound); or the **free drug level** (only the amount of the drug that is not bound to the proteins, which, in the case of carbamazepine, is approximately 25% of the total level); or **the metabolite**, carbamazepine epoxide (which is thought to be an active anti-epileptic agent in its own right). The free drug level represents the medication that is in the blood, but is not bound to protein, that crosses the blood brain barrier and hence is responsible for the effect on the brain. In other words the free drug level reflects the cerebrally active quantity of the drug in the body.

It is important to stress that drug levels are only a help to the doctor in the making of clinical decisions about treatment and are not to be seen as the absolute answer. There is a saying that, **'The doctor treats figures in clothes rather than figures on paper'** and no laboratory result can replace the experience and clinical judgement of a competent doctor. However, I believe in measuring drug levels and monitoring both biochemical and haematological parameters to make sure that the medicines are not causing any unexpected unwanted effects. This is particularly important with DD patients (see Chapter 4) who lack the capacity to report some of the side-effects of treatment and so are unable to protect themselves against iatrogenic (doctor induced) complications of the illness.

Use of monotherapy or polytherapy

There is also debate as to whether one should use only one drug (**monotherapy**) or try drugs in combination (**polytherapy or polypharmacy**). The decision as to which drugs to give in combination is based on an understanding of the type of epilepsy which is best treated by the medications and also an understanding of how the drugs work.

Some drugs work by reducing the amount available in the brain of excitatory neurotransmitter (chemicals that are found in the brain and act between nerve endings to increase brain activity). Other drugs work by increasing the amount of inhibitory neurotransmitter (chemicals that act at the end of nerves in the brain but have the opposite effect to excitation and dampen down brain activity). It is logical to combine drugs which are effective in the same type of epilepsy and which work by different means so that the drugs are complementary.

One should aim at monotherapy and only use polypharmacy if the single drug fails to keep the epilepsy under control.

Can anti-epileptic medicine do harm?

There is no medication that is absolutely free of side-effects or unwanted effects and the patient should always be on the look-out for adverse reactions. Every drug is capable of causing nausea, vomiting, diarrhoea, skin rash and headache. All the anti-epileptic medications are active on the brain; if they were not active on the brain then you would have to question how they could stop the fits. All of these agents therefore can cause problems with thinking, behaviour, balance, tremors and clumsiness. Each individual drug may have its own special problems, such as increase in body hair with phenytoin or teeth and gum problems resultant from gingivitis (gum infections) that are also more common in patients treated with phenytoin. The patient should be aware of these potential problems and report them to the doctor if they occur.

In some situations the medicines can make the epilepsy worse and, again, this should be thought of if such a change in epileptic pattern occurs. Not all doctors will be aware of this possibility and thus it is a good idea to keep it in mind and refer to the doctor any deterioration in the epilepsy when the patient is treated with a new anti-epileptic medication.

The need for compliance

Compliance means following the doctor's advice. There is little point going to see a doctor and not taking the medicines as prescribed. Every person may miss his or her pills from time to time and this is not regarded as being non-compliant, but there is good reason to take extra medication as soon as one realises that pills have been missed. It is productive to anticipate this possibility and to discuss it, in advance, with the doctor so that one knows what to do when the occasion arises. If there is a good reason for not taking the medicine as advised by the doctor then this should also be discussed as soon as possible so that an alternative can be considered. There is no point trying to fool the doctor because, in the end, it is the patient who loses as a result; it is the patient who will have the fit.

The place of epilepsy surgery

Anti-epileptic drugs are the main stay of the treatment of epileptic fits but they are not always effective. In about 20% of cases the fits continue to be frequent, even after trying many different medicines. In these cases it is worth considering **epilepsy surgery**. This is a very specialised area of epileptology and requires the doctor to define the exact place, in the brain, where the epilepsy starts and then to be sure that this part of the brain can be removed without leaving the patient worse off than before the surgery.

The patient needs to be fully assessed, using the range of investigations that were described in Chapter 3. Once the doctor is convinced about the nature and place of the origin of the epilepsy, the patient needs to undergo detailed psychological investigations to make sure that removal of this part of the brain will still leave the patient able to cope.

The patient will have a test, known as an **Amytal Test** (named after the type of barbiturate, amylobarbitone, used in the test) or as the **Wada Test** (named after the neurologist who developed the test), in which the short acting barbiturate is injected into one of the main blood vessels to one side of the brain to see if the other side of the brain can still maintain memory and language. Memory and language are vital to ensure the ability to perform daily functions. Both sides of the brain will be tested like this to make certain that the results are reliable.

Only once the doctor is satisfied that the patient will be able to continue to do routine daily activities after the affected part of the brain has been removed will the patient be referred for epilepsy surgery. The success rate for epilepsy surgery is about 70–80%, assuming that the team has properly assessed the patient and correctly identified the epileptic focus to be removed. Sometimes this proves to be more difficult than one is led to expect and the final decision may depend upon a value judgment based on the odds and probability of success. In these situations it is even more imperative to explain the risks of failure to the patient so that he or she can be involved in the decision-making process. This empowers the patient, or the family, to play an active role in the management of the epilepsy and also prepares people for possible outcomes.

There is another form of epilepsy surgery which does not aim at removal of the epileptic focus because the investigation of the epilepsy has not shown that there is a specific focus to its origin. In these cases it is sometimes felt that division of the cerebral hemisphere connections may reduce the amount of epilepsy by stopping the spread of abnormal activity. In these patients the corpus callosum (the connections between the hemispheres) is surgically divided; the operation is called a callosotomy, it is usually restricted to patients with generalised tonic and atonic seizures, both of which can present with drop attacks. It rarely stops fits but may reduce the frequency of drop‚attacks.

The other surgery performed in epilepsy is hemispherectomy in which a whole hemisphere is removed when it has been shown that the tissue in that whole hemisphere is grossly abnormal and its removal may stop seizures.

Patients sometimes have great difficulty in coping with the eradication of the fits because they have become accustomed to being epileptic and almost enjoy playing the 'sick' role. Having epilepsy allows them to receive special consideration and attention which is lost once the epilepsy is controlled. They cannot cope with control of their fits and this is particularly shown in patients who have undergone epilepsy surgery because this group usually represents the worst affected group of patients who have often had the longest history of epilepsy. Successful surgery may cause very serious psychological problems because of the arrest of seizures, and this should be addressed in the work-up period to minimise these subsequent problems. All successful epilepsy surgery centres can report cases of suicide, or attempted suicide, following successful operations which cured the epilepsy but destroyed the patient.

Do these treatments cure the epilepsy?

It is basically wrong to think that these treatments are cures. What they do is to control the fits in those cases where they are successful. Having said that, it must also be said that, if the person is fit-free for two years or more, there is a 60% chance that, if medication is stopped, they will remain seizure free. If the person remains fit-free for two years after epilepsy surgery, then the doctor may choose to withdraw medication, assuming all other parameters are favourable.

Are there other ways to treat the fits?

Various doctors have tried alternative approaches to treating epilepsy. These include acupuncture, hypnosis, naturopathy or biofeedback, but none of these is as effective as conventional anti-epileptic medication or epilepsy surgery. The general opinion amongst traditional Chinese medicine therapists is that **acupuncture** has very little to offer, although the acupuncture needles are excellent for use as short term sphenoidal electrodes (special electrodes inserted just below the cheek bone and used to perform a particular type of EEG investigation, discussion of which is beyond the scope of this book) when this procedure is undertaken in the doctor's private rooms.

Hypnosis may have a minor role to play in controlling fits in patients who have simple partial onset seizures. By this it is meant that if the person has an 'aura', then they may be able to prevent progression to convulsive fits by means of self-hypnosis.

Hypnosis also has a role to play in **relaxation** of patients whose fits are related to stress. For this situation it could be very helpful to teach a patient self-hypnosis.

It is too early to give much advice about **biofeedback**, but it is fair to say it is not widely used or advocated and that is usually indicative of lack of efficacy. As regards naturopathy, **there is always benefit from eating a healthy well balanced diet** that provides a nutritional complement to daily living. Again, there is little widespread use of naturopathic remedies in the treatment of epilepsy and this is usually taken to suggest that their efficacy is still unproven.

There is another form of treatment that is currently undergoing evaluation and that is **vagal stimulation**. This requires the surgical implanting of a stimulator, which is quite an expensive piece of equipment, by a competent neurosurgeon. The idea is that the stimulator will give impulses that will work to stop fits. It is far from clear how this functions, or if it is worth the cost, but trials are under way and you should know that such techniques are available in case you wish to learn more about them.

There are also those who say that, as epilepsy is an unpredictable illness, it is not possible to be certain that, even if the person stops having fits, the benefit can be assigned to the treatment given. One has almost reached the point where science is taking over from common sense, but it is important to make this distinction, as was already pointed out when looking at the role of the regulators.

Can one ever stop taking the medicine?

Inherent in the last paragraphs was the understanding that, for most forms of epilepsy, if the person becomes seizure free and the EEG does not show gross signs of epilepsy, then the doctor may choose to try to wean the person off medication after about two to five years; this will have a 60% success rate. Scientific literature suggests that this withdrawal of medication should be undertaken even if the EEG is frankly positive for epileptic activity but this is not the option which I follow. I still use the EEG to help me to decide if I am going to stop the medicines. Once the decision has been taken, and again I stress the need to involve the patient in the decision-making process, then the weaning process should not be rushed, but one cannot be dogmatic as to how slowly this should be done.

There are a number of factors that should be taken into account when considering stopping anti-epileptic medications. Some of these suggest a good outcome and others suggest a less favourable result. Those factors influencing a positive consideration of the withdrawal of medications include: absence of evidence of neurodevelopmental abnormalities; earlier onset of epilepsy (onset in childhood); categorisation as one of the generalised epilepsies (excluding some of the secondarily generalised epilepsies such as Lennox Gastaut Syndrome); easy achievement of control with the introduction of medications; a benign seizure pattern, such as in Benign Rolandic Epilepsy. The converse is applied as an indicator of patients in whom it would be unwise to consider withdrawal of medications, without serious discussion with the patient and his or her family, because of the increased risk of further seizures.

Social factors also need to be considered, such as the need for some patients to drive to keep a job. Withdrawal of medication should be accompanied by a period in which the patient stops driving and this may prove to be impossible. A patient may need to drive children to various out-of-school activities and it is unacceptable to subject the children to the risks of a seizure occurring in the weaning trial. Again it can be seen that each case must be assessed on the conditions that are unique to the patient.

Chapter 9

Epilepsy care means more than just treating fits!

Quality of life

The initial treatment of epilepsy has to be directed at stopping the fits but the real aim of treatment, in any condition, is to improve the **quality of life** for the affected person and, if practicable, for those in contact with that person, such as the immediate family, friends, schoolmates or workmates. Quality of life is the difference between what is expected from life and the reality of what that life has to offer. It is a very subjective, abstract commodity and its quantification is the subject of quite extensive research around the world.

Detailed discussion of the science of 'quality of life' research is beyond the scope of this book but this chapter will look at some of the psychosocial factors which are known to impact upon it. Quality of life touches all aspects of a person's life: physical, functional, emotional and economic.

The unpredictability of fits causes its own problems for the affected person. It is often the fear of having a fit in public, and the resulting humiliation and embarrassment, that stops the epileptic achieving maximal benefit from life. People with epilepsy often refuse to go to public places, a refusal which puts a stop to such simple daily activities as catching public transport, shopping, attending sporting fixtures or just going to the movies. It can be seen that epilepsy can greatly inhibit the epileptic's enjoyment of life. Often the epileptic will withdraw from daily activities and deny themselves the possibility of realising his or her full potential.

The child with epilepsy and what to look for

Epilepsy can touch every facet of life from growing up, family life, education, seeking work, marriage and parenting and almost any daily activity. **The child may be over protected by his or her parents** and be denied the right to try the wide tapestry of experience that life has to offer. I have seen a boy refused permission to join the boy scouts; the refusal came both from the parents, who feared that the child may have a fit and injure himself, and the scout leader, who thought that the activities of scouts are too dangerous for an epileptic. In the final analysis, it was fear and prejudice that were the real limitations to the child's right to enjoy life to the full.

There are some commonsense areas where restrictions to the child's life are not only acceptable but are to be encouraged. Such areas include swimming; no child should swim without responsible supervision. This is an area of concern where the ruling must be enforced for the epileptic as well as for the non-epileptic child. Similarly the law now requires that children wear crash helmets when riding pushbikes. Parents should insist on this with all children but especially so with the epileptic child. The same insistance should apply to horseriding, a situation where protective headgear is a necessity.

Some doctors dissuade parents from allowing their epileptic children to have baths because they feel that showers are safer. This may be so, but I am less dogmatic in directives to parents regarding this activity, although it is fair to say that the child having a fit in the bath may drown as a result.

Epilepsy and the family

Other family members are sometimes embarrassed about having a family member with epilepsy. Parents may feel guilt and even blame themselves or, worse, their spouse for passing on the gene that caused the epilepsy. I have seen families that have dissolved because of this guilt affecting the parents' relationship.

Siblings (brothers and sisters) may feel jealous that the epileptic is receiving the lion's share of the parents' attention, or angry that the epileptic is not expected to contribute as much to the daily chores that are so much a part of running family life. Siblings may be embarrassed by the brother or sister having a fit in public. There is sometimes the perception that the epileptic is stupid and that, by association, their family members must also be stupid.

The way the family deals with the epilepsy may have real benefits. If the family can discuss, in depth, the issues that surround the child's epilepsy, and their own fears that are likely to influence the way the family functions, then there is a chance for the family to grow as a result of the experience. It is important that no one in the family feels shame about the epilepsy, and the possibility of this reaction needs to be brought out into the open so that it can be dealt with.

The way that a family deals with a seizure may also be important. It has already been said that witnessing a seizure can be a very frightening experience. **Family members will have the same type of fears as do others, but these may be exaggerated** by the feelings of guilt or shame that have already been described. It is most important that the family be encouraged to deal openly with these feelings and not hide them.

The family should not try to run away from the diagnosis but needs to confront what is part of that family's existence. In the introduction to this book, the person with epilepsy was advised to accept the diagnosis as a matter of fact; it is likewise advisable for the family to treat the diagnosis in the same way. **The acceptance of the diagnosis by the family should be therapeutic.** If the family is accepting of the diagnosis in the same way as the epileptic is, then others may be more prepared to accept it also.

Parents often have less expectation for the epileptic child to achieve in school, sport or activities that are competitive. This obviously reduces the child's competitive edge in life and this will reduce his or her ability to realise maximal potential. The lack of encouragement in childhood will have for-reaching consequences. This failure of the epileptic to achieve can increase the feelings of guilt felt by the parents who, for the best of intentions, have limited their child's capacity to achieve and then have seen that 'failure to realise full potential' affect the child's future development in every facet of life. The need to extend oneself is an important component of a child's overall development.

Adolescent siblings are already vulnerable from distortion of their concept of who they are, and may blame the epileptic family member for any difficulties that they are experiencing in this complex time in their own development.

Adolescents with epilepsy

The epileptic adolescent will have similar problems to those described in the last paragraph and may have to add to these the problem of rejection, not only from outside the family, but even from close family members.

Many of the issues examined in the section dealing with the epileptic child are also relevant to the adolescent, especially the adolescent newly diagnosed with epilepsy. The diagnosis has different consequences depending upon the time in the life of the individual when the diagnosis is made. Adolescence is one of the most vulnerable periods in life. It is the time when self-image is 'coming together' and the individual has to accept the reality of who and what he or she is. Much of the basis of self-image has already been put in place but the new diagnosis of epilepsy has the risk of destroying a 'healthy' self-esteem. It is important that those who come in contact with the newly diagnosed epileptic both help the epileptic to accept him- or herself as well as show the young person that he or she is acceptable to others.

There is a risk that the adolescent may regress and become very childish and dependent upon others such as family and friends. Parents need to encourage the adolescent epileptic to take responsibility for his or her own well-being and to develop the ethos, or attitude, of self-reliance and independence that is so much a part of growing up.

Epilepsy and education

Teachers often also share the parents' reduced expectations for the child with epilepsy and because of this are prepared to accept second-, or even third-best from a student who under other circumstances would be forced to both try harder and achieve more. Because epilepsy involves the brain, it is often wrongly assumed that the epileptic is less intelligent than others of the same age and equal capacity. It is another case of ignorance and mythology replacing fact and reality, but unfortunately perpetuation of the myth can achieve a self-fulfilling prophecy. This means that everyone is satisfied with less than maximal effort on the part of the epileptic child or adolescent and as a result it is reasonable to expect that the epileptic will never do their best.

This general acceptance of failure may then translate into a reduced estimation by the epileptic of his or her own worth. People with epilepsy must be encouraged to achieve maximal potential in life. They should be advised to aim for a career path in which they can be self-employed and to do this most effectively they should seek to achieve absolutely the best that they can in school and subsequent education. I have been challenged as to why I should advocate 'self-employment' and the answer is straightforward. People who are self-employed are somewhat insulated against the discrimination that still exists in the real world; they cannot be dismissed and they are the masters of their own destiny.

Teachers need to acknowledge responsibility to reduce the stigma that may impact upon the epileptic student and to support the epileptic individual in seeking maximal potential. One of the ways this can be achieved, in the classroom situation, is to have the class undertake a research project designed to examine the nature and impact of epilepsy. This will make the class aware of what it means to be an epileptic and will also have the effect of making the epileptic student the only class member who can provide personal insight into the condition and its consequences.

Epilepsy, social interaction and marriage

It has been shown that **epileptics have reduced potential for marriage or forming close relationships** and it is not surprising if, throughout their lives, they have been taught that they are less valuable than others, that they also develop lowered self-goals.

Children are often described as very cruel. They are likely to jibe and ridicule the person who is different, and what could be more different than the epileptic disrupting the rhythm of the class with a seizure. There may be more than one child with epilepsy in the class, but this would have to be the exception rather than the rule, based on the accepted prevalence figures.

As implied above, a teacher has the capacity to use the classroom situation as a positive learning experience to educate the class, producing compassionate and understanding people who could be ambassadors for those with epilepsy. Unfortunately the teacher is also only a mere person and is often guilty of harbouring the same negative attitudes as prevail in the community as a whole. Thus the teacher often misses the golden opportunity that has presented itself.

From the above it can be seen that discrimination against the epileptic starts from an early age. Often epileptics themselves contribute to this discrimination. As stated in the Preface, people with epilepsy react to the diagnosis as if there is justification for denying its presence. They treat it as shameful and refuse to accept that they are epileptic; this contributes to the negative image. This has been discussed throughout this text and will not be revisited at this stage. Suffice it to state that there is need for everyone to change attitudes so that the person with epilepsy can overcome the limitations that are imposed both from without and from within.

The question of sexuality

An important part of social interaction is the very real consideration of sexuality which can be affected by epilepsy in a number of ways. Both men and women complain about **decreased libido**, due to epilepsy. This can be a direct consequence of **negative self-image**, depressed sex drives resulting from not accepting oneself and thus being unable to accept that anyone else could want to have a sexual relationship with an epileptic.

The **anti-epilepsy medications can adversely affect sex hormones** and thus physiologically reduce libido through a purely hormonal effect. It has already been said that these medicines can cause the patient to be sleepy and may cause headache, both of which are unhelpful to an effective sex drive.

Fear of having a seizure during the act of sexual intercourse can act as a very potent reason for avoiding sex and the epileptic may be too embarrassed to nominate this as the reason for avoiding a sexual relationship. This can have all sorts of consequences, ranging from the partner feeling that he or she is considered unworthy, to the partner even questioning the sexual preferences of the epileptic.

The obvious solution to this dilemma is to always have an honest relationship with a potential sexual partner and to ensure open and complete communication. This may have a very positive effect. The partner may feel flattered that the person with epilepsy has taken them into their confidence and may reward such a compliment by being more considerate and accommodating. There is also the risk that the person may show sympathy rather than empathy, and, again, this can be overcome only by honest and complete communication with the partner.

For the epileptic woman there may be a question relating to the use of contraception. It must be remembered that **some anti-epileptic drugs can reduce the amount of the oral contraceptive pill that is available to the body**. This is because anti-epileptic medication may increase the rate at which the liver metabolises the hormones in the pill. It is important that the epileptic woman who is using oral contraceptives, discusses this with her doctor so that supplementary contraception, possibly using physical barriers such as diaphragms or condoms at times of increased risk (such as at the time of ovulation), can be examined and discussed and suitable alternatives organised.

Changes to lifestyle

One final consideration is that social interaction can be directly affected by the **need to change one's lifestyle because of the epilepsy**. For example, **people with active epilepsy are not permitted to drive** and that can seem very restrictive, especially upon a young man who may feel that a woman would not wish to date him if he cannot pick her up and drive her to a social engagement. **Epilepsy and alcohol do not mix well** and a young man may feel that he cannot go to the pub with his friends if he cannot also drink alcohol with them. In both these situations the epileptic must seriously question the type of people with whom he or she is associating if they are unaccepting of even these minor restrictions.

Another restriction that epilepsy may impose results from the fact that some forms of otherwise quite benign epilepsy may be very badly affected by sleep deprivation. Thus, the epileptic with this type of epilepsy (typified by Juvenile Myoclonic Epilepsy) may be forced to leave social functions earlier than his or her peers and this might create friction with friends. If friends have been chosen with wisdom then this should not cause too much of a problem but, again, it can challenge the person's perception of self-worth. It can also make the epileptic feel even more 'different' and add to the person's perception of stigma.

Stress can also adversely affect epilepsy but it is almost impossible to avoid stress in modern fast living. I believe that it is inappropriate to advise the epileptic to avoid stress because to do so would mean to avoid competition or challenge and that would make it impossible for the epileptic to realise their maximal potential. There are some measures that can be taken to diminish the amount of stress that the epileptic must endure but it is important that such interference with lifestyle does not reduce capacity to have maximal quality of life.

One of the ways to deal with specific situations of stress is to use minor tranquillisers before such recognised and anticipated and predictable times of stress. An example of this is the use of a minor tranquilliser before a particular patient embarks upon a sporting activity known to provoke fits. If this means of situation control is contemplated, it may be necessary to ask for prior approval from the sporting body's governing authority to avoid prosecution for illicit use of drugs. Even so, approval may be refused.

Marriage

With social isolation it is to be expected that the epileptic will have less opportunity to meet that special person with whom he or she would like to spend the rest of life. It follows that the prospects for a happy marriage are somewhat reduced for the epileptic as compared with those for the general population.

As suggested earlier when examining limitations on social interaction for the epileptic, because of decreased self-esteem the epileptic may see him or herself as unworthy of the love and support that is a vital part of any marriage. Reduced self-esteem may mean that, even if the epileptic meets Mr or Ms Right, they may lack the confidence to 'follow through'. It can be seen that there are a number of reasons why the person with epilepsy has lower expectations for a rewarding marriage.

The role of self-help groups

As shown above, social interaction is an aspect of life in which the epileptic condition can have a very negative effect. **Self-help groups can fill the void.** They can give the affected person social contacts, the feeling of belonging and the realisation that he or she is not alone. There is also the potential to contribute to the organisation and so improve one's self-esteem by doing something felt to be worthwhile.

Each self-help group will be different and the character of a single group will change with time because the membership is usually quite fluid. It is not a criticism of the group that members come and go, but rather a result of the changing needs of the individual over time. It is a general experience that the individual will be an active member of the group until certain needs are met, and then the person may well move on. Depending on the vitality of the group, that member will be replaced by someone else whose needs may be quite different and thus the goals and objectives of the membership may change with time.

The structure of some of the groups has become more complex and, as a result, **some self-help groups have employed 'professional' administrators**. This can be highly beneficial, with greater advocacy and lobbying at government level. A greater range of services can be developed along with more professional delivery of counselling and consideration of vital issues such as employment, training or education. Unfortunately it can also be a destructive move because the administrator may be out of touch with the epileptics, who comprise the membership, and may choose to restrict delivery of services.

The choice of which group to join must be answered on an individual basis after the prospective member has had the opportunity to have a good look at the structure and activities of the body under consideration. Each person's needs and expectations will be different, as are the various self-help groups, and it is only with careful scrutiny that the best selection can be made, benefitting both the epileptic and the group.

If there is any doubt about the structure of the group or the benefit of joining it, then it may help to discuss this with other epileptics or even with the doctor who should be well equipped to advise each individual patient according to special needs and expectations.

Employment and epilepsy

Employment is an area that is greatly reduced for the epileptic. As a rule of thumb, **any job that requires the wearing of a uniform is denied to the epileptic**. This may seem a somewhat radical statement, challenging much of our current dogma which denies the presence of officially condoned discrimination, but its truth will be apparent as you read on. Just stop to consider the types of work that require the wearing of a uniform. They include driving public transport, serving in any branch of the armed forces, the jobs of police officers, firefighters and airline pilots and many of the romantic occupations that growing children imagine to be the ultimate in achievement and which are publicised by television and the movies. Basically these jobs are denied to the person with epilepsy. **Despite the law against discrimination on the basis of physical impairment, epileptics often report experiencing significant discrimination** and reduced ability to find work.

In routine practice it is my approach to advise patients to seek to be self-employed. While governments can legislate to eliminate discrimination, this is an unrealistic exercise because it is impossible to legislate to change attitudes. Only with commitment to education can anyone expect to change attitudes. There is evidence to suggest that attitudes are changing but it is a slow process and will need a lot of commitment from many people before there is the acceptance of epilepsy that the affected population so desires.

One cannot ignore that there are real occupational safety considerations to be taken into account when addressing the question of employment for the epileptic. Work at height, or work with dangerous machinery, is not advisable for the epileptic, for his or her own safety. The safety of others is also a consideration. There are a number of jobs which immediately come to mind as unsuitable, such as taxi driver, heavy transport driver or surf lifeguard.

Epilepsy and travel

There is no reason why someone with epilepsy should not be allowed to enjoy travel and the wonders of our ever shrinking globe. There are a few considerations that do need to be taken into account. These include accommodation of the changing time zones which may cause patients to miss doses of medication and it may be helpful to discuss this with the doctor before travelling. Patients also worry about taking drugs through customs checks and it has been my policy to provide patients with a letter identifying the medications that the patient is taking and the regimen in which they take them. If provided with sufficient notice, I will also often write ahead to colleagues overseas to advise them that one of my patients will be travelling in their corner of the globe, just in case the patient has a problem while there.

It is prudent for the epileptic who is travelling to avoid the excesses that may accompany travel, such as lack of sleep, taking excess advantage of the free alcohol provided by well-meaning airlines and the need to see and do everything to avoid missing out. Prudence recommends taking out suitable travel insurance and I have often completed medical questionnaires for my patients to ensure that they do gain access to appropriate cover. Some insurance companies are better than are others and epileptics should shop around for the cheapest and most comprehensive cover, recognising that they have a pre-existing condition. It is worthwhile discussing this both with doctor and travel agent to ensure the optimal result for all concerned.

Epilepsy and domestic chores

Just as it may be dangerous for the epileptic to operate some forms of machinery, so cooking, especially with an open flame, may pose risks, especially for the person with uncontrolled seizures. Modern cooking appliances, such as microwave cooking, may offer suitable alternatives. Some modern cookers also use convection or fan-forced cooking which is reasonably safe and cost efficient. Use of slow, crock-pot cookers for soups and stews is economic and safe. Appliances with pre-set timers may overcome the problems of spoiling food because a fit occurs during meal preparation.

Other domestic jobs, involving the use of equipment such as lawn mowers, electric edgers, power tools (such as drills) or chainsaws, may pose risks which are unnecessary and in certain circumstances it may be better to seek help rather than place oneself in a dangerous situation. As with so many aspects of daily life, common sense must be used to assess the degree of acceptable risk.

Epilepsy and recreation

There are recreational pursuits, such as scuba diving, hang-gliding, sky-diving, abseiling, rock-climbing or bungy-jumping, which are not to be considered for the epileptic. It follows that any occupation related to the teaching or practising of these pursuits is also out of contention for people with epilepsy.

Some recreational activities, like some areas of employment, have established minimal standards of physical fitness for participation. Examples are driving a racing car, even as an amateur, or flying a plane, even one's own aircraft.

Epilepsy and driving

People with active epilepsy are not allowed to drive any form of motor vehicle. The main exception to this rule is the epileptic who only has 'nocturnal' seizures (fits experienced only during sleep, rather than specifically at night) and has had only such 'sleep related' fits in the past 3 years. The other exception to the ban on active epileptics driving is the case of the person who only has what many call 'auras', although you now know that these are simple partial seizures in which consciousness is not impaired.

Obviously there cannot be any restrictions imposed on the epileptic who is not yet aware that they have epilepsy and thus a quarter of the population of people with active epilepsy is still driving, blissfully ignorant of an epileptic condition. There is a push by various bodies around the world to establish a universal code regarding driving restrictions for those with epilepsy. Classifications for the proposed code are active epilepsy, semiactive (seizure-free period has been less than 5 years but longer than, say, 1 year) or inactive (seizure-free period is the mandatory 5 years). The inactive epileptic is usually allowed to drive private vehicles; for the semiactive epileptic restrictions still vary according to where he or she lives and who manages the epilepsy; and the situation for active epileptics has already been discussed.

The rules also differ according to whether the person holds, or held, a driver's licence at the time that the epilepsy was diagnosed or whether they have had a single major convulsive episode or a series. As we enter the age of enlightenment there seems to be emerging a general consensus that is allowing each case to be considered on its merits and the input from the attending specialist medical practitioner is playing an increasing role in the final determination of what restrictions are to be imposed. In my own practice I hold to the rule of thumb that the person who has had uncontrolled epilepsy is restricted from driving for a period of approximately 12 months in which they must be seizure-free before I will complete the necessary documents required by the driving authorities. I still believe that one cannot be overly dogmatic and each case needs to be considered on its merits, but I offer this as an indicator of my standards. I am not aware of any case in which I felt that the patient should be eligible to hold a drivers licence, based upon the advice from the patient concerning the control of his or her epilepsy, but in which the local driving authorities over-turned my decision and refused to grant the licence.

I have had a case in which the patient lied about the control of his fits and I based my decision to endorse his application for a drivers licence on that false information. The patient killed an innocent pedestrian as a result of a seizure while driving, and it was only after this that it was clear that the patient had lied about his seizure control. In this case the patient was found guilty of manslaughter and spent 9 months in gaol. I endorsed this conviction and the need to ensure honesty between the doctor and patient. This incident raises serious questions regarding the responsibility of doctors to report those patients whom they believe pose risks to the public and about the whole question of compulsory reporting. It is likely that, had I realised that the patient was still fitting, I would have increased medications to stop the fits and the patient may have then been able to drive legally without the obvious risk and without an unnecessary death. I have seen the patient since his release from gaol, and, if he is to believed, he is now seizure-free because of a change to his treatment. Again, each case needs to be considered on its merits but this case highlights what can go wrong when there is a lack of honesty and trust between doctor and patient.

Epilepsy and pregnancy

Women with epilepsy, when they become pregnant, may have an altered risk of seizures. The statistics broadly suggest that the expectant mother's epilepsy becomes worse in about 40% of cases, improves in about 10% of cases and is unchanged for about 50%.

It is not clear what the use of anti-epileptic drugs means for the unborn baby but there are some recognised risks for teratogenicity (risk of malformation in the unborn babe). Examples of this include the risk of spina bifida with maternal use of valproate, and the well-reported 'phenytoin syndrome' in babies born of mothers treated with phenytoin. In this syndrome the baby may have cleft lip and palate with abnormalities of the hands and heart. Similar features to those of the phenytoin syndrome occur in the offspring of mothers who take carbamazepine.

If an epileptic woman plans to become pregnant, she should discuss these plans with her doctor before she becomes pregnant. Once she knows she is pregnant it is usually too late to do anything to protect the fetus (unborn baby). By the time she finds out that she is pregnant she is usually well into the first 3 month period of the pregnancy which means that the damage that could occur has already happened or, alternatively, it is not going to happen.

With the newer generation of drugs, either developed or being developed, the effects in pregnancy are unknown and because of this these drugs are contraindicated in pregnancy. Most drug trials clearly exclude any woman who is not practicing reliable contraception, or who is breast feeding, so as to protect the fetus, or the baby (as well as protecting the company from being sued by the mother or offspring should a disaster occur).

If the doctor fears that a female patient is less than reliable with contraception, then it is worth considering the prescribing of folic acid for this patient as it has been shown that use of folic acid protects the fetus from spinal malformation. It is unclear if a fit (especially a major tonic/clonic convulsive episode) during a pregnancy badly affects the fetus, but it seems reasonable to assume that it would be better for all concerned if such a fit did not occur. The biggest risk of fits occurs either in the early part of the pregnancy or at the time of giving birth.

I have adopted the standard approach that it is unwise to give too much medication in the first trimester (first 3 months) and if possible to avoid increasing dosages in this period. To protect all concerned I only chase drug levels in the last trimester (last 3 months) to try to stop fits during the actual birth process because no-one needs the extra stress of a fit at that time and it is a time of increased risk of seizure.

Epilepsy and breast feeding

Women often become anxious about being on medication while they are breastfeeding. (The process of forming breast milk is called lactation.) As it is basically the free fraction of a drug, namely the unbound part of the circulating medicine which is not attached to the blood proteins, that gets into the breast milk, it is only a very small percentage of the anti-epileptic medication that is passed on to the baby in the case of most of the commonly used medicines. The other fear is of having a seizure while feeding the baby and it is wise to take whatever precautions are available, such as feeding the babe in a protected environment. An example of this might be to feed the baby while propped up in the middle of a double bed, or, if the epilepsy is less well controlled, to feed the baby in a comfortable position sitting on the floor with pillows around to protect both mother and baby should a fit occur. It is unwise to feed the baby while walking around, for fear of dropping the infant if a seizure occurs during the feeding.

As with so many issues in the care of the epileptic and family, it is important to use common sense. Breastfeeding usually requires night feeds and this may cause sufficient sleep deprivation to increase the rate of seizures. If this is the case it may be necessary to consider bottle feeding so that the father can help with night feeds. Some mothers are lucky enough to have their own mothers to offer a helping hand in the demanding time. So long as the involvement of another person does not create too much stress in the household it might be worthwhile accepting the offer of help during the time that breast feeding is required, especially if there are other children in the house who also need supervision. It is a pity to be too proud to accept help when help is really needed.

A final comment should be made to protect the mother from feelings of guilt should it be impossible for her to breastfeed. Stress and fear may interfere with the production of sufficient supplies of milk for the baby and it is wrong to add this consequence to any burden of worry. If the baby is not gaining enough weight, or there are problems, this situation should be discussed openly in the family and with the doctor. To every problem there is a solution.

The epileptic parent

After the over-protection of their own childhood it is reasonable to expect epileptics to make similar mistakes in the parenting of their own children. With reduced self-esteem and lack of drive to achieve maximal potential it follows that there is great room for inadequacy in being a parent. There is grave danger of the epileptic parent being too timid to encourage his or her children to fully realise the opportunities in life.

The parent with epilepsy is sometimes too self-conscious about the condition to even tell his or her own child about it and may conceal the diagnosis. This may mean that the first time the child realises that the parent has epilepsy is when witness to the parent having a major tonic/clonic convulsive fit.

This can be very frightening and has the possibility of undermining whatever relationship existed between the generations. Such lack of confidence between parent and child, also serves to emphasise the negative attitudes that surround epilepsy and may suggest to the child that the parent is a less valuable person as a result of the epilepsy.

Failure to disclose epilepsy to family and friends indicates lack of trust. It suggests that the epileptic cannot even trust 'mates' to be supportive, and re-emphasises the issues raised in the preface to this book. It indicates that the epileptic, the person most likely to know what it means to be epileptic, perceives that being epileptic is a shameful state and it follows that if he or she sees it as such (and he or she should know the truth) then it is so!

The need for regimentation

It is easy to overlook the very intrusive nature of epilepsy, even allowing for good seizure control and a compliant and realistic patient. Epilepsy dictates that the affected person needs to be fairly regimented to take medication at prescribed times and in prescribed quantities. The epileptic is dependent upon the doctor to provide the optimum in patient care, and thus needs to have a good doctor/patient relationship. As already set out above, being epileptic may mean that the young person does not go to the pub with his or her friends because alcohol and epilepsy do not mix well. People with juvenile myoclonic epilepsy must get sufficient sleep to protect them from having further fits. These restrictions illustrate the extra need an epileptic has for disciplined attitudes.

In an era when taking drugs is seen as indicating weak character, the person with epilepsy is dependent upon drugs to live a full life. This may mean that they are seen as less valuable than their friends or associates. Epilepsy and water sports are seen as an area of risk for the epileptic, yet swimming is an integral part of the young person's life, especially in a country like Australia. Expertise in water activities and surfing are seen as measures of virility for the young male, and as a great social outlet for all involved, but the person with epilepsy is dependent upon friends to keep an eye on him or her while in the water. This reduces feelings of independence and means that the young epileptic is not free to do things without the consent of others.

Some people with epilepsy are subject to fits if exposed to stroboscopic lights, set at certain frequencies of flash. This means that some young people cannot go to discotheques with their friends and hence feel socially isolated. This particular form of photosensitivity can even interfere with the epileptic's enjoyment of computer games such as Star Wars or other such games which involve rhythmical flashing lights, and can reduce the person's use of computers in daily life. Only about 10–15% of people with epilepsy are prone to photoconvulsive seizures and thus this constraint only affects a very small number of epileptics.

The restriction on driving for the person who only has one fit a year seems most unfair to the epileptic but it is important to protect others in the community as well as the epileptic. It is hard for the young to accept some of the restrictions that epilepsy places on their daily routine. Transportation is seen as a significant part of social interaction and the denial of a drivers licence and the lack of mobility and social intercourse that this restriction imposes reinforces the dependence that is epilepsy.

It can be seen that epilepsy has the potential to touch every aspect of the epileptic's life and the doctor needs to offer a holistic approach if he or she wants to treat all the issues that epilepsy provokes. What has been set out in this chapter are just some of the many and varied effects that epilepsy can produce. These provide food for thought so that both the doctor and the patient can prepare to discuss them in more detail and so that you are again provoked to think about the issues that are epilepsy and how these affect the epileptic person.

Chapter 10

Summary. Where to from here?

Objective of the book

In this book I have tried to introduce you to the complexity that is epileptology and to indicate the areas in which debate and confusion still cloud our knowledge. The aim of the book has not been to provide the ultimate text book on epilepsy; that would be an unrealistic objective. The book has aimed at whetting your appetite and hopes to be the catalyst encouraging you to go beyond what is included here and to read further.

Definition and classification

Chapter 1 defined what epilepsy is and made the point that the development of epileptology has seen the evolution of two different classifications, namely the ILAE classification of seizures and that of the epilepsy syndromes. This has meant that research is internationally interchangeable. Having said that, it must be remembered that any classification is only as good as the person using it and thus the applicability of these classifications is determined by the level of knowledge and experience of the doctor involved. The important point to remember is that epilepsy is no longer just a single entity but rather a complex collection of differing phenomena. This breadth of differentiation has relevance to the choice of treatment and the predictability of prognosis.

Differentiation was extended in Chapter 2, to give the reader a basis for discussion of differing approaches to treatment. Epileptic fits and the epileptic syndromes are broadly divided into focal and generalised, depending on the site of origin of the epileptic activity. Standard treatment was noted as divided in a similar way into carbamazepine for partial seizures (usually part of focal epilepsy) and valproate for generalised fits (found in generalised epilepsies), but treatment of epilepsy was not covered fully in this chapter.

Diagnostic process

Chapter 3 explored the way that epilepsy is diagnosed. The point was reinforced that the most important tool in the definition of the diagnosis is obtaining a clear history and a description of what actually happened during a seizure. Everything else is of secondary importance and, even if all other tests are negative, if the history and description of the epilepsy is convincing then the diagnosis is established.

The most useful test in epileptology is the EEG and Chapter 3 set out the variety of EEG investigations that are available to help the doctor decide on the diagnosis. The EEG has more use than just confirming the diagnosis as it is also used to help decide which part of the brain is the origin of the epileptic activity. Chapter 4 discussed other investigations, such as MRI, SPECT or PET scanning, all of which are used to better define both the anatomical and physiological activity of the brain, both between seizures and at the time of a fit. Chapter 5 examined what to do in a variety of seizure types.

The need to look beyond the epilepsy

The point was made that it is insufficient to diagnose that a person has epilepsy; this addresses only half of the question that the epileptic wants answered. The person wants to know why he or she has epilepsy and Chapter 6 discussed the genetics that are involved in the passing on of the epileptic gene from one generation to another. This chapter made the claim that all epilepsy has an inherited threshold but that this is lower for the person who is diagnosed as being epileptic compared to that for the average person who does not carry the label. One of the messages of this book has been that it is easier to label a person as having epilepsy than it is to remove the diagnosis if it was wrongly applied.

Chapter 6 also examined the causes of epilepsy and the need to define the cause so that this could be addressed and, if practicable, treated; the patient may not then be committed unnecessarily to a lifetime of medication. An example where this approach is applicable is the need to stop the alcoholic from drinking alcohol rather than treat the epilepsy per se.

Epilepsy look-alikes

There are a number of conditions that can be misdiagnosed as epilepsy and Chapter 7 was devoted to examining these and providing clues to protect the naive from making diagnostic mistakes. These conditions include pseudo-seizures, syncope and vaso-vagal episodes. It is very important that the doctor has excluded these before the patient is labelled as an epileptic.

New and exciting treatment for epilepsy

In Chapter 8 the treatment of epilepsy was discussed with attention directed both at the currently used medications and the newly developed drugs, not all of which are yet released for general sale at the pharmacy. You have been provided with my perspective as to the relative merits of these newer agents. The role of epilepsy surgery was considered and the necessary tests discussed. The question of monotherapy versus polytherapy was reviewed with a preference noted for monotherapy initially. For situations where monotherapy fails, the approach of rational polypharmacy was considered, with emphasis on the necessity to align the mode of action and the scope of efficacy with the type of epilepsy being treated. The mode of action should be complementary so that the epilepsy is addressed from as many aspects as possible (for example, by using agents which enhance the dampening down of activity within the brain by decreasing neuro-excitation and increasing neuro-inhibition, working by means of complementary neuro-transmitters).

The need to address all aspects of the patient's life

Chapter 9 dealt specifically with what is perhaps the most important issue in the treatment of any condition, the need to improve quality of life for all concerned. Epilepsy causes significant restrictions for both the epileptic and those with whom he or she comes in contact. Issues such as dependence on drugs, altered lifestyle with limitations on mobility, recreational pursuits, employment potential, educational stimulation and basic questions of social intercourse were analysed. Highlighting these factors, which can so negatively impact upon a person's daily life, provided you, the reader, with food for thought; it is not always obvious that a condition, such as epilepsy, can so restrict quality of life. Once these issues have been recognised, then you can do something about them and ensure that they do not destroy a person's life.

A look at the future

What remains is to consider ways in which the future for those with epilepsy can be improved. The drug companies are spending a fortune looking for new and better anti-epileptic medicines and improved ways of testing how they work and proving their efficiency. Governments are passing laws to reduce discrimination and doctors are becoming more aware of the need to provide holistic medicine and to treat all aspects of the patient's life. Society is becoming more accepting of epileptics, at least on the surface, and the future seems more positive.

Books like this are designed to encourage you to look beyond the superficial and to educate yourselves about epilepsy. Education is the backbone of the future for people with epilepsy. It is important that epileptics accept themselves and as a result stand up to be counted. At the opening of this book the point was made that epileptics are their own detractors when they give the impression that to be epileptic is to be less than acceptable.

If this book has encouraged epileptics to be more accepting of themselves and, even more important, encouraged both epileptics and their associates to read more and to become better educated about epilepsy in general, then it has done its task. The time has come for epileptics to be their own ambassadors and to go out and educate others. It is time for epileptics to take responsibility for their own future and to fight for a better deal.

Throughout this book you have been invited to read more about epilepsy and have been asked to send any comments, generated by reading this book, to me. You are seen as a valued partner in the production of a book designed to meet the needs of the person with epilepsy, his or her family and friends. Only with constructive criticism can the optimal text be produced and that has to be the goal of anyone trying to educate.

I conclude by thanking you for taking the time to read this book and I also thank you in advance for taking the trouble to contact me with any suggestions that you may have for improving its worth.

Glossary

Absence seizure Primarily generalised seizure in which the person suddenly stops what he or she is doing and will be, as the name implies, mentally absent and out of contact with the world.

Action potential The tiny electrical impulse that travels down a nerve carrying its message along the axon.

Agranulocytosis A disorder characterised by extreme reduction or even complete disappearance of the neutrophils in the white cells of the blood. This causes loss of resistance to infection which may allow sepsis and death.

Atonic seizures Primarily generalised fits in which there is uncontrolled overactivity of the brain causing a loss of muscle tone.

Aura Often falsely thought to be a warning of a fit which is about to happen. This is a simple partial seizure.

Axon The arm extending from the neurone, the nerve cell, that allows the nerve to send its message to other nerves or muscles or glands.

Biofeedback A technique used in psychology, training a person to recognise certain states within the body, such as tension or an impending seizure.

Callosotomy Dividing the corpus callosum, the bundle of fibres which allows connection between the two halves of the brain, known as the cerebral hemispheres.

Catamenial epilepsy Epilepsy which is related to the menstrual cycle and hormonal changes, either at the time of ovulation or menstruation.

Cataplexy A state associated with narcolepsy. When the person has a cataplectic episode he or she collapses at times of emotional excitement such as times when jokes are told or he or she is upset.

Classifications Established to provide internationally agreed standards and to make an acceptable tool for both clinical management and research use. The ILAE has established two different classifications within epileptology, the international classification of seizures and the classification of syndromes, in 1981 and 1989 respectively.

Clonic seizures Primarily generalised seizures in which the person has repeated muscle spasms but the amount of movement is less dramatic than in myoclonic fits; the repetitive nature of the jerking is more pronounced and of longer duration than in myoclonic seizures.

Cognition Thinking, intellectual activity, ability to do psychological tasks of reasoning, calculation, visual and spatial orientation, reading and writing.

Complex partial seizure A focal fit type in which there is impairment of consciousness but the focal nature of the fit is maintained.

Compliance Doing what the doctor has ordered, which in epilepsy usually means taking medicines at the doses and frequency prescribed.

Computerised tomographic scan (CT) A cerebral imaging technique which uses X-rays plus sophisticated computer technology to produce detailed images of what the organs look like and an idea of the anatomy of the structures in the head.

Cryptogenic Of unknown cause.

Deja vu The feeling that a person has done the thing before or has been through the experience before. It is the result of a false memory or of an uncontrolled overactivity of the memory area of the brain.

Dystonia Abnormal posture adopted due to abnormal muscle tone.

Electroencephalograph (EEG) A technical tool recording the small electrical discharges which represent the activity of the brain.

Enteric coating A special cover around tablets or capsules to delay disintegration until they have passed through the stomach and into the small intestine. This causes slower absorption and may cause less gastric side effects.

Epilepsy A tendency to recurrence of seizures.

Epileptic The adjective from the word epilepsy. 'Epileptic' is often used to indicate a person with epilepsy and does not imply any form of insult or derision.

Epileptology The study of epilepsy.

Fit This is the same as seizure — see Seizure.

Focal seizure See Partial seizure.

Frontal lobe epilepsy A type of focal, anatomically defined epileptic syndrome in which the patient may show very bizarre behaviour.

Generalised seizure See primarily or secondarily generalised seizure.

Generic A broad name to cover a group of like items. In the pharmaceutical industry a generic reference is to a medicine or drug by its approved name rather than by a specific tradename for the drug as produced by a particular company. For example, phenytoin in England is known as Epineutin while in Australia it is commonly known as Dilantin. Both Dilantin and Epineutin are tradenames for the generic phenytoin.

Gilles de la Tourette A condition associated with tics (unusual brief movements of the muscles) and grunts, sniffing, snorting, the tendency to repeat what was just said (like an echo) and a compulsive urge to swear and use bad language.

Grand mal This is an out-of-date term used to describe a major tonic clonic seizure. It is often used to suggest a primarily generalised convulsive fit though in reality it is more likely to be a secondarily generalised seizure

Half-life The time taken for a compound to be reduced to half the original amount; a term commonly used in nuclear medicine and pharmacology.

Heavy snorers syndrome A condition in which the patient snores excessively, arousing suspicion of sleep apnoea.

Hemispherectomy Removal of a badly damaged brain hemisphere in special types of epilepsy.

Hypersomnia Excessive sleepiness.

Hypnagogic myoclonus A feeling as if about to fall off a cliff, experienced just before drifting asleep. Hypnagogic means falling asleep and, for myoclonic, see myoclonic seizures.

Iatrogenic Brought about by something that the doctor has done.

Idiopathic Of unknown cause of illness.

International Bureau for Epilepsy (IBE) An international umbrella body which represents the various national organisations made up of the non-professional (self-help/lay) bodies dedicated to improving the image of people with epilepsy, at both national and international levels. Unlike the ILAE, this organisation is concerned specifically with non-medical groups in the struggle to help people with epilepsy.

International League Against Epilepsy (ILAE) An international umbrella body with various chapters representing the different countries where there are professional organisations for epileptologists.

Isotope A radio-active compound used in nuclear medicine and injected into the patient to create images as seen in SPECT or PET scanning.

Jamais vu Opposite of Deja vu, this is a feeling that the familiar seems foreign. This too is potentially epileptic in nature.

Juvenile myoclonic epilepsy A type of generalised epilepsy syndrome which is characterised by myoclonic fits, particularly prone to occur if the person has late nights, excess alcohol or is non-compliant with medication.

Lennox Gastaut Syndrome An epileptic syndrome which occurs more commonly in children, but also in adults. It includes generalised tonic seizures, myoclonic seizures, tonic/clonic seizures and may also include atonic seizures plus both simple absence and atypical absence seizures. It is associated with a special EEG pattern and is usually very difficult to treat. It is associated with intellectual problems (usually retardation with developmental delay) and a poor prognosis.

Lesionectomy A surgical procedure in which the abnormal tissue thought to cause the fits is removed.

Libido Emotional craving, usually sexual, which promotes activity to satisfy need.

Lobectomy Removal of one of the lobes of the brain, usually the temporal lobe.

Magnetic encephalograph (MEG) Measures the tiny magnetic fields that go with the brain's activity. This is still mainly a research tool.

Magnetic resonance imaging (MRI) A technique using large powered magnetic fields to produce photographic images of the brain by means of special computer technology and recording procedures.

Monotherapy Treatment with only one type of medicine.

Myoclonic seizures Primarily generalised fits associated with sudden forceful muscle jerks or contractions. The limbs (more commonly the upper limbs) are flung out without control in a wing-like fashion.

Narcolepsy Also known as a sleeping sickness because the person can fall asleep at almost any time. It is associated with very quick onset of 'rapid eye movement' sleep (known as REM sleep) which causes vivid hallucinations as sleep overtakes. Also associated with cataplexy, sleep paralysis (in which the person will lie in bed and feel paralysed until touched by someone) and somnolence at almost any time if not fully stimulated to stay awake.

Neurologist A specialist physician trained in illnesses of the nervous system. The category is now further divided into various subspecialty areas such as 'epileptology', 'strokology', 'parkinsonsology', newly coined words denoting specialist areas in the management of each of these illnesses. Category also divides into neurophysiologists, who study how the nervous system works, and clinical neurologists who treat patients presenting with sicknesses of the nervous system.

Neurone A nerve cell.

Neurotransmitter The substance that is produced by a nerve cell allowing it to send messages across the small gap, between nerve cells, called the synapse. Neurotransmitters can be excitatory or inhibitory, e.g. GABA which inhibits the activity of nerve cells, and glutamate which excites responsive neighbouring cells that come into contact with it.

Nocturnal seizures Fits that only occur during sleep. In epileptology the term 'nocturnal' relates to 'sleep' rather than time of day, Shift workers can have day-time 'nocturnal seizures'.

Paediatrician A doctor specialising in the study of illnesses of children.

Partial seizures Focal onset seizures. Partial seizures are divided into simple and complex partial seizures plus secondarily generalised seizures.

Periodic limb movement in sleep Also called periodic leg movement or restless leg syndrome. A condition in which sleep is interrupted by excessive leg movement.

Petit mal An outmoded term often incorrectly used to mean 'a small fit'. Correctly applied the term denotes a primarily generalised absence seizure.

Photosensitivity A cause of reflex epilepsy in which the patient responds with seizure to particular stimulation by flashing lights. It affects approximately 10–15% of epileptics and may be provoked by computer games.

Physician In some societies the term just means a doctor, but in anglo-saxon medical tradition it implies a medical specialist, as distinct from a surgeon.

PLMS See periodic limb movement in sleep.

Polypharmacy See polytherapy.

Polysomnograph A test performed in a sleep laboratory in which bodily functions, such as heart function, brain function, sleep-staging, limb movements, oxygen dispersal in the blood, breathing and snoring are recorded and evaluated to look for sleep disorders.

Polytherapy Use of more than one type of medicine when treating an illness.

Positron emission tomography (PET) A sophisticated imaging technique that uses a medical cyclotron (a machine which makes radioactive compounds) to make short half-life isotopes (radioactive compounds). These substances are injected into the patient and nuclear medical imaging is used to map out the metabolism, or receptor sites, in the brain depending on the nature of the substance injected.

Prevalence The number of cases of a particular condition that exist in a community. It is the ratio of those with the condition within a set number of the community, (e.g. x [the number of cases of the condition]/100000 of the population).

Primarily generalised seizures Fits which are generalised from their onset and are divided into: absence seizures; myoclonic seizures; clonic seizures; tonic seizures; tonic/clonic seizures; and atonic seizures. In each of these fit types there is no definable focal onset to the fit.

Projection The meaning depends upon context. In neurophysiology, the projection of the nerve is taken to mean the range of transmission of the nerve's message. In psychology, projection is the transference of an emotion onto someone else, so that an angry person perceives the anger as directed at him or her from another rather than originating inside him or herself.

Pseudoseizures Episodes that look like seizures but do not come from 'uncontrolled overactivity of part or all of the brain' but rather have a psychological basis.

QOL See quality of life.

Quality of life The difference between what is expected from life and the reality of what that life has to offer. It is a very subjective, abstract commodity and assessment of it aims to quantify the enjoyment that life has to offer.

Receptor sites Specialised areas in cells (including brain cells) which bind to chemicals such as neurotransmitters and drugs. Different receptor sites are specific for structures on particular chemicals. Interaction between receptor site and chemical causes a particular response in the body.

Reflex epilepsy A form of 'situation related epilepsy' that is provoked by a variety of stimuli, such as photic stimulation which causes fits as a result of stroboscopic flashes of light. Most commonly experienced with the lights in a nightclub or computer games or television.

Refractory Resistant to treatment; the prescribed medicines have failed to control the epilepsy.

Schizophrenia A mental/psychiatric illness involving difficulty with thinking and keeping thoughts restricted to a single topic, involving feelings of ambivalence (uncertain and mixed feelings towards situations or people) and associated with hallucinations which may be confused with epilepsy.

Secondarily generalised seizure Convulsive conclusion of the spread of brain activity which started as a partial seizure. In the secondarily generalised seizure, the focal nature of the fit is replaced by involvement of the whole of the brain and this causes the person to have a convulsion.

Seizure The expression of uncontrolled overactivity of part or all of the brain.

Signs Clinical findings resulting from the physical examination of the patient and documented by the doctor.

Simple Partial Seizure Focal onset fit that is not associated with impairment of consciousness and can progress to complex partial or secondarily generalised fit.

Single photon emission computerised tomography (SPECT) An imaging technique which uses nuclear technology but uses chemicals more stable than those used in PET and thus does not need a medical cyclotron on site. It uses special nuclear medical cameras to record pictures of the brain, and maps out the way the brain uses blood (which is called the perfusion of the brain). The parts of the brain that are using more blood are assumed to be more active at the time of injecting the isotope rather than at the time of scanning.

Sleep apnoea Stopping of breathing during sleep, either due to obstruction of the air passages (obstructive sleep apnoea) or from central causes in the brain (central sleep apnoea).

Somnambulism Sleep walking.

Spastic In the neurological sense of the word, a pathological increase in muscle tone.

Status epilepticus Prolonged seizure or little or no time between repeated seizures. If allowed to continue status epilepticus can cause death or irreversible brain damage.

Synapse The minute space that exists between nerve cells. This space requires neurotransmitters, rather than electrical impulses, to carry the nerve's message from one cell to another.

Syncope Medical term for a faint.

Symptoms Complaints reported by a patient when the doctor takes a medical history.

Syndrome A collection of features which appear together. Medically, denotes a collection of signs and symptoms that in combination are foundation for a diagnosis, an absolute understanding of the reason why these symptoms should appear together is not implied.

Telemetry See video-EEG

Teratogenicity Risk of malformation in the unborn babe as a result of the mother taking medications during the pregnancy.

Therapeutic window The reported range of a drug, as measured in the blood, which controls a condition (say, epilepsy) without causing side effects. Based on analysis of a population sample.

Tonic fits Primarily generalised seizures associated with sudden spasms of the muscles, for example of the arms which may become stiff and be held out in front of the person.

Tonic/clonic seizures Primarily generalised convulsive fits. It is this type of epileptic fit that was called Grand Mal before the new classifications were accepted.

Vaso-vagal attack Faint produced by excess stimulation of the vagus nerve causing a sudden drop in blood pressure and a decrease in the blood supply to the brain resulting in loss of consciousness.

Vertigo An unreal sensation of motion not caused by movement but sensed as such.

Video-EEG The patient is connected to an EEG at the same time as they are being video recorded so that the doctor can see both the brain activity and what the patient is doing at the time of the so called fit. This is also called video-telemetry because it sends the signals to a recording station which may be in a room, separated from the patient, where the technician or nurse can observe the patient.

Video-telemetry See video-EEG.

Volt A unit of electromotive force which is produced by 1 ampere of current carried against 1 ohm of resistance. A technical term used to indicate the amount of electricity provided by the electrical system that operates in any given location, for example, 110 volts in America or 240 volts in Australia.

WADA test Barbiturate is injected into one of the main blood vessels to one side of the brain, to see if the other side of the brain can still maintain memory and language. Both sides of the brain will be tested like this to make certain that the results are reliable.

Withdrawal seizures Fits which occur as a result of suddenly stopping taking medicines or other agents, such as benzodiazepines barbiturates, alcohol.

Index

113